Praise for Keep It Off

Kristie's book KEEP IT OFF is a no-nonsense approach to reducing unwanted pounds. Her energetic attitude, diet Pepsi in hand, is a style of achievement that will have you feeling as if Kristie's right there with you every step of the way cheering you on, 'You got this!' Change your mind, change yourself, change your weight! I recommend her book for anyone struggling to maintain a healthy weight.

–*Robert B., Bestselling Author*

Kristie's book KEEP IT OFF is a powerful story filled with resilience and honesty. She's not sharing her journey to hear, "Wow, I'm so proud of you!" - she's sharing it to show you and everyone that everything is possible, even during the toughest times. This journey is proof that perseverance works. Kristie radiates unique energy and passion, which I've witnessed during Zumba classes! I wholeheartedly recommend this book - it will make you laugh, inspire you, and most importantly, give you hope.

—Diana Munoz Coronado. SSW and Zumba Fitness Instructor

KEEP IT OFF is relatable, even humorous at times, inspiring, and motivating. Kristie's desire to reach and help others in their weight loss journey is evident in her writing. She allows herself to be vulnerable as she shares her triumphs and setbacks with the hope that even just one person will benefit from the journey she has made as she accomplishes and maintains her desired weight. Truly worth your time. Read it (warning...not on an empty stomach)!

—*Kim Holm*

KEEP IT OFF is an excellent reflection of choice everyone makes in day to day life. Kristie has done an amazing job in sharing her journey. Initially it sounds easy to hear that she lost 100 pounds, but when you read this book you will realize and understand that it is not easy, it's a journey of over two decades and a choice she made every single day and how she programmed herself. I love the way she has written with humor. It keeps the reader engaged and wanting to read the next chapter in anticipation of what will come next. I am not a book reader, but I completed this book within 5 days as I felt Kristie is talking to me in person and narrating her story, I know Kristie is a great storyteller and you can realize that in this book. The way she has narrated the various situations I am sure it will motivate anyone to be active and pursue their goals irrespective of they are looking to reduce their weight or not.

–Swapnil Amrutkar

Copyright © 2025 by Kristie Williams

All rights reserved. No part of this publication may be reproduced, distributed, or transmitted in any form or by any means, including photocopying, recording, or other electronic or mechanical methods, without the prior written permission of the publisher, except in the case of brief quotations embodied in critical reviews and certain other noncommercial uses permitted by copyright law.

ISBN: 978-1-7349568-2-5

Front cover image by Forest City Publications

First printing edition 2025

Forest City Publications
9972 Cattleman Rd
Holbrook, AZ 86025
Lara@forestcitypublications.com

Keep It Off

How I lost 100 Pounds and
Kept it Off For Good
(And How You Can Too!)

Kristie Williams

Contents

Praise for Keep It Off	1
Contents	6
Acknowledgements	9
Introduction	12
Green Beans, Ice Cream, & Pizza	13
Apples, Pears, & Celery	32
More Salsa, Less Chips	42
Grilled Chicken & Diet Pepsi	56
Keep Saying No to the Oreos	67
Endless Highway	72
Cheese Fries & Samosas	89
Sweet & Spicy	94
Don't Let Go of the Wheel	115
Protein Shakes & Rainbow Nerds	159

Plan…& Then Stick to the Plan	169
Time to Get Started	202
Things that Inspire Me	230
Diary of a Foodie	235
My Heroes	250
Case Studies	259
Keep Going, Keep Coming Back	274
About the Author	277
Suggested Books & Businesses	279

To my son Sean

Acknowledgements

Robert Bautner, my friend and mentor, who spent countless hours with me on this project and continues to inspire me in so many ways. Thank you for your friendship, your guidance, your never ending positivity.

Sean Williams, my one and only kiddo, whose formation and arrival motivated me to start my journey to become the best possible version of myself.

Denise, my only sister/sibling, my first best friend, my confidant, thank you for all the laughs, tears, special moments, eye rolls, sarcasm and meme sharing over the past 50+ years. Thank you for being there for me always. I love you very much!

To Eric, Dad, Cathy, Mom, Steve, Amanda, Nathan, and the rest of my family and friends spread across the US: I love you all. Thank you for being such an important part of my life.

Edie Peterman, my best friend for over forty years, who has been cheering me on the whole way, thank you for your continual everlasting friendship and support.

    Cirilo Albino DeJesus (Joel, Bear), my closest friend, hiking buddy, bucket list crushing travel buddy, food loving eating buddy, concert going buddy, home and car repair specialist, thank you for everything you have done for me and brought to my life the last 10 years. Words cannot express my appreciation.

    Wade Baldwin, Diana Munoz Coronado, Cirilo Albino DeJesus and Samantha Madsen, first thank you so much for your friendship and support in so many ways for so many years. Secondly thank you for sharing your experiences with me and allowing me to include them in this book.

    Diana Munoz Coronado, Kim Holm and Leigh Pearson, my guinea pigs (beta readers LOL). Thank you for agreeing to read this book and share your thoughts with me. I can't wait to get your feedback!

    Lara Helmling, my editor, publisher, friend, words cannot express my gratitude for all the time, effort and support you have given me and put into this project to make it a reality. Thank you!

My Zumba Family–Arcy Leon Corona, Erika Leon, Julia Leon, Mama Leon, Diana Munoz Coronado, Ruben Coronado, Rocio Diaz, Irvin Juarez, Beto Montero Rodal, Christopher Santana, Erika Beltran, Eva and Oscar Galvan, Ana Lopez and so many more the list goes on and on. Thank you for accepting me, welcoming me and making me feel like one of the family in every single class. Thank you for your energy, choreography, music and fun. I can't get enough!

Swapnil Amrutkar, Kim Holm, Humberto Rodriguez and Sagar Soni, my coworkers and friends that I talk to every day. Thank you for always having my back, supporting and encouraging me at work and in life..

Samantha Madsen, my friend and fitness instructor, I have already said so much about you in the book itself. You are just an incredible person and I can't thank you enough for everything you have taught me by your example for so many years in so many ways.

To the long list of those not called out above, sorry I ran out of space! :-)

Introduction

Imagine for a moment sitting with your best friend, any friend, casual acquaintance, coworker or a complete stranger in their living room, kitchen, a restaurant, the airport or anywhere and the conversation you would have. What would the topics be? Now meet me, Kristie Williams, an open, outspoken, caring, energetic, passionate, never shy, not afraid to discuss any topic with anyone, woman who has been on a weight loss and fitness journey for over 20 years. I've lost 100 pounds and kept it off for over 14 years and I would love to have a conversation with any of you, all of you, about any topic, not just weight loss and fitness. This is my story and I want to share it with you!

Green Beans, Ice Cream, & Pizza

My story started long before I knew there would be a story to tell. When I look back on my relationship with food, many things come to my mind. Growing up, my mom was never a foodie. She still isn't. She has always been ridiculously thin as far back as I can remember. For many years and even now, she has the opposite problem of everyone I have ever known–she can't gain weight! I usually say, 'there's a problem I would love to have'…but maybe I wouldn't. I often tell her I could help her gain weight, as to me it is super easy. My dad is for sure a foodie. At every holiday, he would pile up his plate with samples of every kind of food available, including every single dessert. He just loves food. Many people do. Honestly, I think it would be sad not to love food, considering how often we have to eat. I think he learned about eating and food from his parents and I from him. I've always believed people grow up emulating what they see. This can be fortunate or unfortunate. For me, it was unfortunate.

Most of my early memories about food revolve around spending time with my family. We built our relationships over lots of delicious food. All except one time. I call it the green bean incident. Let me preface this by mentioning that my eating habits were/are quite unusual. I didn't like any vegetables, any fruits, fish, and most condiments. When I was about five years old, my dad told me not to leave the dinner table until I ate a green bean. I was at the dinner table for at least two hours. I finally ate the green bean. I immediately threw up and haven't eaten a green bean since. My dad never asked me to do that again. I think he gave up.

I remember going out for pizza as a family–my parents, my sister and me. It felt like we would sit at the Pizza Gallery forever. My dad has always eaten so slowly, and back then he wouldn't drink anything until he finished eating. After he drank his soda, he would smoke a cigarette. This was back in the day when restaurants had smoking sections. We would sit and wait impatiently for all of this to transpire before we could leave.

I remember my mom making cakes for birthdays out of the Betty Crocker cookbook. One cake she made for me was shaped like a cat with chocolate cake and chocolate icing of course as chocolate is my favorite for all desserts. It had whiskers, eyes, nose, etc. One cake she made for my sister looked like a gingerbread house except it was white and had life savers on it. My sister has never been a big chocolate person so her cake and icing were vanilla.

When my parents had an argument, the whole family would go to Dairy Queen for ice cream. My mom would always get the peanut buster parfait. The rest of us would get cones (always chocolate for me), and my dad would eat the curls off the tops of all of them! My dad has always loved ice cream and I suppose taught us to use it as a way to deal with disappointments in many situations. Can't afford the car you want, let's go get ice cream! I never saw it as a way to soothe pain or resolve problems, but it sure did make you feel better immediately after a disappointment or just because.

I remember spending a lot of time with my grandparents on my dad's side. Oh how I loved them. I

Keep It Off

still miss them so much. They had a huge impact on my life and the person I am today. As soon as you walked in their door, my grandmother and/or my grandfather would ask if you wanted something to drink and eat. That's what a good host/hostess does, right? In my family, the sign of a good day, event or celebration starts and ends with being fed. Food was the measure of a good life. My grandfather always had a jar of nuts next to his chair, mainly peanuts or cashews, and a hunk of sharp cheddar cheese in the refrigerator to share with us. They always had ice cream in the freezer, too. We looked forward to eating all that good stuff every time we visited. And that was in addition to whatever meal we were going to have.

> In my family, the sign of a good day, event or celebration starts and ends with being fed.

We had a lot of pizza and spaghetti at my grandparent's house. One time my uncle was there. I remember because he asked if there was milk. He announced that he couldn't eat spaghetti without a tall glass of milk. I thought that was weird and funny at the same time.

My grandfather used to cook big delicious steaks back when they didn't cut the fat off and they weren't so expensive. My grandfather cooked us breakfast a lot, primarily pancakes using his special mix, with sausage on the side. One time we went camping with my grandparents and my grandfather decided to make pancakes. It was my two cousins, my sister and me. One of my cousins was the only boy. My grandfather asked him how many pancakes he wanted. He said he would have two if they were good. He ate fourteen!

We went camping with my grandparents a lot. We would have hot dogs and polish sausages over an open fire on a long two pronged fork. We had as many marshmallows as we wanted. We would go to an Amish farm store, Maplehofe, to get fresh eggs and chocolate milk. They had homemade ice cream and we would all get a cone and sit in the front of the store in handmade chairs and swings, eating our cones. Sitting in the camper or at my grandparents house the conversation would go like this: at breakfast, grandfather would say to grandmother, 'what are we going to have for lunch?' At lunch, the question was, 'what are we going to have for dinner? At dinner, he asked, 'what are we going to have for dessert? And what about tomorrow for breakfast?'

From this you can probably tell that my grandfather was the force behind our eating habits. From the time I can remember, he was overweight, but my grandmother was not, which is interesting looking back on things.

I remember spending a lot of time with my aunt, uncle and two cousins when I was growing up. My uncle would take the lid off a half gallon of ice cream and grab a spoon. He would pour cereal in a serving bowl, add milk and keep the box there with him. He could and still can eat an entire large pizza by himself.

For holidays, there was always an over abundance of food. Mashed potatoes were and still are the most beloved food and by nobody more than my uncle. He has always made a mashed potato volcano! He is still teased to this day. Someone inevitably says, "You better get in line for the potatoes before your uncle does," and someone else chimes in, "Are there any potatoes left?" "How many pounds did you make this time?" The usual amount is 10-15 pounds. I swear under my family crest, it should say, "If it tastes good, keep eating!" We've had tons of family events over the years–bridal showers, baby showers, birthdays, anniversaries, weddings, holidays, game nights, barbecues, and volleyball games. These are the same two questions for every event: 'What do you want me to bring?' and 'What are we going to eat?'

There was always so much yummy food. Always so much overeating. While my parents were still together, my sister and I participated in a few activities–twirling batons and playing softball. We also used to play outside a lot, riding our bikes, so we kept active and thin. I remember after our softball games, my dad would take us to 7 Eleven and let us pick out some candy and get a small slurpee.

This is how I was raised. This is how I learned to eat. After my parents got divorced, I lived with my dad for a while and my sister lived with my mom. I remember my dad cooking sloppy joes. We would sit on the couch and eat Hydrox cookies while watching

Keep It Off

TV (we couldn't afford Oreos I guess and they tasted better anyway). I stayed thin because I still had gym class at school doing arm circles, jumping jacks, mountain climbers, etc, and anywhere I wanted to go I walked or rode my bike.

When I was thirteen, I went to live with my mom and sister. We lived in an apartment complex. In the summer we would live at the pool and at night play a tag-like game called 'Relievio.' For breakfast I would have Dr. Pepper and peanut butter flavored TastyKakes every day. For lunch if I had money I would get school lunch, usually pizza if they had it. My mom often worked two or three jobs and wasn't home much at dinner time. It became normal not to have any food in the house. I would open the refrigerator to find only a pitcher of ice water and maybe a 2-liter of Coke or Dr. Pepper. If there was food to eat, I would cook for me and my sister, usually instant mashed potatoes or egg noodles with brown gravy. Sometimes my mom would scrape the bottom of her purse for a couple dollars or some change and my sister and I would walk up to the shopping center and get a slice of pizza at Chat n' Chew. Sometimes if we had a little more money, we would get subs from Country Maid. Other times my mom would bring something home from The Big Top Deli where she worked. I went from always having money or food available or a meal with no question, to not knowing one day from the next if there would be anything to eat, money to buy anything or if there was food, being responsible to prepare it.

When our family was together, food was a HUGE part of our lives and all events and it was a sign of happiness and fulfillment. So many things changed in my life at this time and it wasn't really a stable strong home environment to thrive in. I believe this was the start of my overeating and weight gain as when food was available and I didn't know when it would be again, I overindulged all the time. As a result of the divorce and circumstances, I was parentified at thirteen years of age.

Before I was fourteen, I started doing a paper route and babysitting kids in the apartment complex. I would use the money I earned to buy candy and junk food and I would eat it all at once. One day my sister and I got in a fight and she said I was fat. She was right and it was only the beginning. When I was fifteen and still in high school, I got working papers so I could get a job. I got a job at the Hot Shoppes travel plaza on I-95 in Delaware where people could stop and get a snack, a fast food meal at Roy Rogers, or a sit down meal at Bob's Big Boy.

    I worked at a snack bar that served chocolate chip cookies, popcorn, ice cream, coffee and sodas. Sometimes if I didn't have a ride, I would walk there from the high school. Fortunately, I got a discount on food and when I got my break, I would go over to Roy Rogers and get a cheeseburger with cheese on both sides, French fries and a Coke. I worked there for three years, moving from the snack bar to the gift shop, filling the vending machines and finally in the office doing paperwork.

    When I was sixteen, I got my driver's license and my dad bought me a mint-green Ford Pinto. He said it was robin's egg blue, but that's another story. No more walking or riding my bike everywhere. No more gym class. No more exercise of any type. Now I drove everywhere, so it was lots of trips to McDonald's and similar places. I started to gain more weight, but I didn't pay too much attention to it. I was getting ready to graduate from high school. I had skipped eleventh grade and went straight to twelfth.

By the time I was seventeen, I decided I was fat and needed to do something about it. I started taking Dexatrim and trying to significantly reduce my food intake. On the day of graduation practice, I took Dexatrim and only had a cup of chicken noodle soup all day. I refused to wear shorts because I thought I was fat. It was about 100°F with close to 100% humidity and I was wearing jeans for graduation practice. I passed out cold on the football field and had to be taken in a golf cart up to the office. About this same time, I started to suffer with IBS (irritable bowel syndrome) although that's not the name they gave it at the time. It always presents the same way–I wake up with pain in my stomach, my stomach inflates and gets hard, and I am doubled over in pain all day. Nothing helped for years, but now lying on my stomach and breathing for ten minutes or more sometimes offers relief. I have been to many doctors, taken several tests, tried several diets and medications, but there is no way to anticipate when it will happen or what causes or triggers it.

It still happens. I currently take prescription medication, many dietary supplements, drink a lot of water, walk and exercise daily, but it continues to happen. Thankfully, when I wake up the next day the episode is over. Sometimes there are months between episodes, sometimes just weeks or days. I wish we could figure out what causes it to happen. Is it stress? Something I'm eating?

I've often wondered if my regular diet, if that's what you want to call it, causes it. I mentioned that I didn't eat any fruits, vegetables, or fish as a child. I still don't. I've tried many things over the years– bananas, cantaloupe, broccoli to name a few. I don't like them. The smell of peas when cooking makes me gag. The smell of fish and the feel of fruits and vegetables in my mouth makes me instantly gag. I keep trying different things. I know it's weird, but I can't help it. I do like the flavor of fruits, just not the consistency. These days, I will eat lettuce but only in a salad (not on a sandwich) with cheese, croutons, and dressing. Maybe add an egg in there, but that's it.

Nothing else. I will eat salsa and spaghetti sauce only if it's blended and not chunky. The only exception is potatoes, but do they even count? When I eat waffles, pancakes or French toast, I add butter and no syrup. When I eat hot dogs or hamburgers, I prefer them plain with no ketchup or mustard. When I eat sandwiches, there is no mayonnaise. I don't drink coffee, tea or orange juice. So I guess I survive on meat, carbohydrates, water, and Diet Pepsi.

I say it's a texture thing, but it's really much more than that. If it smells bad, tastes bad or feels weird in my mouth, I'm not eating it. I'm the only one in my family like this. My mom, dad and younger sister eat just about anything. My mom and sister eat a lot of vegetables and fruit. Gastro issues or not, I doubt I could ever eat like they do. Not going to happen.

We did a contest/experiment at work several years ago when we were having a potluck dinner. I worked with this guy from India that didn't like scrambled eggs and I didn't and still don't like bananas. We decided that he would bring me a banana and I would cook him some scrambled eggs. We would see who could eat it without gagging or hurling. I'm not sure who won the contest, but if you could have seen the faces both of us made while attempting to eat something we didn't like! It was hilarious or it is now. There are pictures of it somewhere. I don't remember why he didn't like scrambled eggs, but I do not like bananas because they are so mushy and feel weird in my mouth.

My Adult Relationship with Food Blossomed and So Did My Behind

After I graduated from high school, a friend helped me get a job at Discover Financial Services and over thirty-seven years later I'm still there. From 18 to about 26, I ate whatever I wanted and really didn't pay much attention to the weight I was gaining, my diet or exercise. I did join Gold's Gym once, but only went a few times. I did bowl in a league and helped my dad coach a young girls softball team, but my eating was awful. People always talked about feeling so full, but I seemed to be able to eat a massive quantity and not feel full. People said they wouldn't be able to eat much if they drank a lot of water or other drinks, but I seemed to be able to eat a big meal even if I drank a lot. Every day for lunch, I would get takeout such as cheeseburger, fries and a large soda. For breakfast, maybe a bag of Cheez-Its or a bagel with cream cheese and a bottle of soda. For dinner, I might cook or get pizza, cheesesteaks, or Chinese. No matter what I had, I would always eat it all or go back for seconds. These were my eating habits during the work week. Weekends were even worse. I would eat donuts, ice cream, cookies, potato chips, lots of cheese fries and Chicken Alfredo. On Sundays, I would cook French toast, fried potatoes, sausage and eggs. Two ladies at work said things to me that I have never forgotten: 'you are always so active.' 'I don't understand how you are overweight.' 'You are so determined and dedicated, I can't believe you haven't mastered your weight.' They were right but didn't see me eat.

> If I'm moody, give me foody.

    When I was around 26, I tried and failed at many things. My apartment complex had a small gym, and I went there to try the weight machines and treadmill, but I wasn't motivated and didn't know what I was doing. I joined Weight Watchers and Curves

Keep It Off

twice with people I worked with, but I was inconsistent, didn't improve my diet much, and, unsurprisingly, saw no real results. I tried phentermine and B-12 shots, but again didn't really change my diet much. I tried SlimFast shakes which are supposed to be meal replacements, but I wasn't really successful reducing my food intake. I quit all of these things because my head and heart were not ready. I wasn't in the right place and time with myself.

    I remember driving cross country with my future husband and stopping each day to do some sightseeing along the way. One of our first stops was the Grand Canyon and I was so excited to see it. We got out of the car to walk to the overlook to see the Grand Canyon and I was sweating profusely, breathing heavily and I thought to myself, 'wow there are so many places you want to go and things you want to see. How are you going to do that if you can barely walk a few feet to an overlook at the Grand Canyon?' Although I could partially blame the elevation as I lived at sea level, the truth was it was my weight and lack of physical activity and I knew that. This was a defining moment for me although it would be a couple years before I would really start my journey. This moment and event was in the back of my mind.

I remember one time I was at a drugstore buying something when I was about 28 and the cashier smiled and said, "When are you due?" I said, "Excuse me?" And she repeated, "When are you due?" It dawned on me that she thought I was pregnant! I said, "I'm not pregnant. I'm just fat."

I was able to lose about 20 pounds right before I got married at 28. I got down to 180 pounds. Did I mention I'm 5 foot 1 inch tall? But after the wedding, I slowly gained back all I had lost plus five additional pounds and then I got pregnant at 30 years old weighing 205 pounds.

A Blessing in Disguise

I was pregnant at 30 years old, weighing 205 pounds at 5 foot 1 inch tall and diagnosed with gestational diabetes. In hindsight, this was my blessing in disguise. I had to avoid sugar, watch what I ate and see a nutritionist while pregnant. Thank God for this because I only gained 7 pounds while pregnant and my son weighed almost 8 pounds when he was born.

Keep It Off

Because I had gestational diabetes, they planned to induce labor a week before my son was due. I had a choice of 7/12 or 7/13 and although I do not consider myself a superstitious person and since I was given a choice, I decided not to have my son on Friday the 13th. Since I had gestational diabetes while pregnant, I couldn't have food or drinks with sugar so I told my dad after I delivered, I wanted a Nestle Crunch candy bar and an ice cold Pepsi. He brought me both, but somebody wasn't feeling well while I was in labor and ended up with them, but that's another story! As soon as my son was delivered and they cut the cord, he turned blue. I barely got to hold him and he was whisked away to ICU. He had to be intubated and when they took us to see him he had cords and tubes hooked up all over. He was not expected to live. He was transported via ambulance that same night to A.I. duPont Hospital for Children in Wilmington, Delaware. The next day when he was less than 24 hours old, he had open heart surgery because he was born with a heart defect. I stayed with him in the hospital for five weeks, never going home. The hospital there is wonderful for patients and their families.

Coincidentally (and thankfully) my sister worked across the street from the hospital. Every day while we were there, she would have lunch with me. She would bring food or get something from the cafeteria. My lunch was delivered to the room and I always had the same thing–chicken tenders, mashed potatoes with gravy, a soda and a chipwich ice cream. After a very difficult 12-week maternity leave, it was time to get ready to return to work. I couldn't get back into my size 18 pre-pregnancy clothes and I thought this is it! I have to do something right now! I don't care if I have to look like a sausage crammed into these clothes–I refuse to go up to a size 20. Also, even post-maternity, my sugar levels were too high. They say if you have gestational diabetes and you don't change your diet and start exercising you will become diabetic within five years and I was diagnosed with pre-diabetes. I had watched my grandfather suffer with diabetes for years and I did not want that to be me as a 31 year old woman and new mother. My son was born Thursday, July 12, 2001.

Apples, Pears, & Celery

Everybody wants to have an hourglass figure, but most of us are overripe pears or apples on steroids. Before I lost the weight, I was like the blueberry girl in Willie Wonka after she eats the gum. Now I'm more of a celery stick. What I learned is that all of these comparisons lead us to criticisms, mostly self-criticisms, and that leads nowhere. I was on an author retreat recently and what struck me was how we don't see ourselves the way others see us. The way we see ourselves is so often much much worse than reality. Instead of worrying about this stuff, I had to get down to business and just start doing the work. For me, that meant Weight Watchers and learning to love exercise.

Weight Watchers and Learning to Exercise

My head and heart were finally ready and aligned. I was really serious this time and was going to make it happen! I didn't know when I started, like my job at Discover, how long it would go and I really wasn't thinking about it then. And so, my journey begins. I joined Weight Watchers and Curves for Women again at 32. My original goal when I joined Weight Watchers was to lose weight. I didn't really have a specific amount or magic number in my mind when I started. Weight Watchers helped me set some small starting goals and celebrate each one in increments of 5 pounds starting at 5, 10, 15, 20 and then 10% of my total weight which for me was 21 pounds, and I took it from there. Weight Watchers encourages you not to try to lose more than 2 pounds a week. Slow and steady wins the race! This is a lifestyle change, not a temporary diet. You don't want to lose a lot too quickly and then revert back to your old bad habits. Weight Watchers teaches you to make better food choices by calculating what your daily point count should be based on your gender, age and current weight, and assigning a points value to each food or drink based on calories, saturated fat, sugar and protein.

    This is the method I use, although the program has changed many times over the years and continues to evolve. The Weight Watchers formula has evolved over the years, but the concepts are the same. You can eat whatever you want as long as you stay within your daily point allotment. I get 30 points per day. If I use 20 points on a piece of chocolate cheesecake or two slices of pepperoni pizza (which I have been known to do on occasion) I only have ten points left for the rest of the day. It's a budget. Don't cringe!

On the other hand, if I eat nine ounces of grilled chicken and two eggs, I've only used 10 points and have 20 left for the rest of the day. The best advice I can give is to track your points or whatever you are doing in whatever way works for you. Online, in your head, on paper, etc. It will help you hold yourself accountable, reflect on days where you did great and bring to light areas to focus on improving. Weight Watchers also teaches you about portion control and what serving sizes are supposed to look like. I am old school in so many ways even though I work in Business Technology. I choose to write everything down to do my tracking of food and drinks. I do count out a portion of say pita chips, use the palm of my hand to figure out what 3 ounces of meat looks like, my thumb up to the first knuckle to figure out what a tablespoon of something is, along with other tricks I've learned along the way. I log everything I eat and drink every single day, even if the point value is zero such as water and Diet Pepsi. I do my best to stay within my daily point value. I track as the day goes.

I know it sounds painful or tedious. It really doesn't take that long and I've just made it part of my daily routine. I track other things also in the same place/tracker. I track my weight. I'm kind of obsessed with the scale. I get on every morning after using the bathroom naked and after my shower. I record the lower of the two numbers. I track my weight to gauge how I'm doing. I get on the scale before I go to my exercise class and before I go to bed.

Sometimes I get on the scale before I eat a meal or to help me decide if I can have dessert. I track my exercise and points I earned for the exercise. I plan to walk a minimum of 5 miles per day. I go to an hour long Zumba class at least 4 days a week. On weekends I try to be as active as possible. I hike whenever I get the opportunity. You can trade your earned exercise points for food, but I usually don't. I really track my exercise to make sure I am continuing to be active and the frequency. I track if I have used the bathroom each day because I've had an ongoing issue with that. I track if I had an IBS episode or not. I track if I'm having my menstrual cycle or not because that can impact so many things such as a temporary five-pound weight gain.

You can track whatever is important to you. I've basically been following the same Weight Watchers plan for over 20 years. At the beginning, when you are paying for Weight Watchers, you are expected to get weighed, pay and attend a meeting weekly. My goal back then was to weigh less than the week before. Was I always successful? No! I have been known even to this day to do anything for a good weigh-in. Take off all jewelry, go without undergarments or socks, etc. Whatever it takes, I'm willing to do it. Now that I'm a lifetime member of Weight Watchers, I only have to weigh-in once a month. I can go any time in the month and I don't have to pay as long as I'm not more than 2 pounds over my goal weight and I don't have to attend the meetings.

The meetings are great if you need motivation or encouragement, to talk about your successes or struggles or to get tips or recipes. I've never really gotten much out of the meetings. I've always been a self motivated person. I have been known to go for my weigh-in on the last day of one month and the first day of the next month (2 days in a row). I've been known to go spontaneously any day in the month when I like the number. I've been known to go immediately before a special event and to wait as long as possible to go after a special event. Think holidays, birthdays, etc. Anything to keep

> Don't half-ass anything. Whatever you do, always use your full ass.

my motivation and not get discouraged. When I started Weight Watchers I was 205 pounds. I initially set my goal weight at 160, but when I got there, I decided I wanted to keep going. I decided to set my Weight Watchers goal weight to 125, to allow for a little wiggle room and sustainability (10 pounds give or take) as I set my personal goal to 115.

    Let me tell you, 115 was a stretch goal. I didn't think I would ever see it. I swear I weighed 122 forever and it seemed like no matter what I did with eating and exercising the number would not budge.

Keep It Off

Then I got COVID and lost my sense of taste and smell as well as my appetite. I saw 111.9 on the scale for the first time ever and kept going. The lowest I've seen and one time only is 105.8. The past couple of years I have primarily fluctuated between 108-113. Now I'm wondering if I should change my personal goal to 105? I mean does anyone want to hear that I've lost 92-97 pounds? Wouldn't it be way more awesome to be able to say I lost 100 pounds?

Weight Watchers has taught me so many things such as don't deprive yourself, but at the same time consider if you really need the entire piece of chocolate cheesecake or could you be satisfied with a few bites? Don't keep things in the house that you can't resist or control yourself with. I can't keep chocolate chip cookies in the house. They call to me and I will eat them until they are gone. You have to figure out what you are willing and unwilling to give up and tweak as you go. When I first started Weight Watchers, I drank regular Pepsi starting at breakfast in a massive volume and hardly any water. I learned very quickly that if I wanted to eat actual food and not drink my daily points, I was going to have to make some changes. I switched from regular Pepsi to Diet Pepsi. What a painful process that was, Diet Pepsi has no sugar and no calories. I still drink a lot of Diet Pepsi every day. It took a long time to get used to the flavor and aftertaste. I also used to eat a bagel with cream cheese for breakfast during the work week which was about half of my daily point allowance, not leaving many points for lunch and dinner.

    I shopped around for something quick and easy to replace my bagel and ended up with cereal bars which are less than half the points I was spending on a bagel with cream cheese. I stopped eating things that are high in points except on special occasions, such as Chicken Alfredo, cheesesteaks, cheese fries, regular potato chips and while it was hard at first, I really don't miss any of these things now. I figured if I planned about 6 points for breakfast that would leave me 12 points for lunch and 12 points for dinner and I follow this plan to this day. I replaced regular potato chips first with Ruffles fat free chips and then Stacy's naked pita chips, candy bars with individually wrapped Dove milk chocolates, butter or margarine with spray butter except on French toast, vegetable oil with canola, olive oil or cooking spray. Breaded chicken with grilled chicken, ranch dressing with Italian.

There are so many possible trades you can make. Some work, some don't. Does anyone remember Snackwells or 100 calorie snack packs? Do they still sell those? The picture on the box and the actual size of the snacks wasn't even close and they didn't taste very good. There will be things you are willing to give up or swap and things that you aren't. I pretty much gave up alcohol all together. I was never really a big alcohol drinker anyway. I've never been able to acquire a taste for most of it. Most of it tastes terrible to me so why spend my points or calories on it? Beer yuck. There's a story here, but bottom line I will never drink beer again. All wine I've smelled or tasted reminds me of what you dip eggs in to color them for Easter (vinegar)!

Chocolate may be one that I never fully give up. I've cut back a lot, but oh how I do love chocolate - ice cream, cheesecake, double chocolate donuts, double chocolate muffins, Dove or Godiva, cake, brownies, cookies, etc. I also have to admit that I may have an addiction to Rainbow Nerds, I like to crunch on them while I work. They are sweet, crunchy, full of sugar and terrible for me. I tell myself that crunching on Rainbow Nerds keeps me from eating in between meals and from exhausting my daily points allowance. Then there's Diet Pepsi. These are the three things I'm not sure I will ever fully be able to give up. I've cut back a lot and tried to quit several times, but so far unsuccessful. Quite honestly, I'm not pushing myself too hard on these three things. I've lost almost 100 pounds and kept it off for 14 years and counting. Maybe it's okay not to give up everything? I tell myself everyone has their vices. Mine could be so much worse.

More Salsa, Less Chips

After I lost about 40 pounds on Weight Watchers, I hit a plateau and decided it was time to get some consistent physical activity into my program. I've heard from books, articles and people in variations that for any weight loss program 80% is about what you eat and 20% is exercise. I decided I wanted to lose weight and be physically fit. So, I joined Curves for Women again, but this time I committed. Curves recommended that you go 3 days a week. Remember as I tell this, I was just beginning my physical fitness/exercise journey!

To make sure I got there with no excuses I would pack my gym bag the night before, put it in my car and go immediately after work. I learned if I didn't do this, I wouldn't end up going! I would say things to myself like let me just put in a load of laundry or hang out with my little dude for a couple minutes. Curves was closed on Sundays, so I planned to go Monday, Tuesday and Wednesday to get it over with for the week (that tells you where my mind was and what I was thinking about exercise at the beginning) and also in case I missed a day, I still had Thursday, Friday and Saturday to get my 3 days in. Curves didn't stay open very late - 6 or 7 pm and sometimes I would get held up at work and not be able to make it in time to do a workout before they closed. At the time, I also had no desire to exercise on Friday or Saturday, but I would if I had to to meet Curves recommended 3 days. I never went more than 3 days in a week. I would only do the bare minimum at the time.

There were many things I liked about Curves. The entire workout was 30 minutes with machines to work different muscle groups and recovery boards in between. All the machines and recovery boards were in one big circle, you switched every 30 seconds and you went all the way around twice. The goal was to do as many repetitions on each machine in 30 seconds as you could and then to walk or jog in place for 30 seconds in between each machine on the recovery boards. It was a great place to start a fitness program if you were out of shape and/or overweight. Most of the people there were older ladies, but I didn't care. Some of the other things I liked about Curves besides the minimal commitment of 30 minutes 3 days a week versus other mainstream gyms were: it was women only so nobody was there with their makeup, hair, nails and fancy workout clothes trying to be cute or pick someone up. No men were checking you out or looking at you in a way that made you feel uncomfortable and you didn't have to waste any time waiting for a piece of equipment to become available. As long as there was a machine or recovery board open, you could start your workout.

> So when we order delivery from Mexican restaurants, how does the endless chips and salsa work? Do y'all come back in 20 minutes or do we have to call?

Also, with all the equipment in a big circle all the ladies would be facing each other so you could talk and socialize. Anyone that knows me, knows I love to talk! I met some pretty incredible ladies at Curves. One of them, I'm still friends with today. I went to

Curves for about 15 years until they closed about 7 years ago. I started in Delaware and it was one of the first places I went to transfer my membership when we moved to Utah in 2008. I wanted to make sure I maintained my commitment as soon as possible after we moved. Again, no excuses! I don't know if there are still places like Curves out there today? I always thought it would be a great place to return to when I'm older and my body can no longer handle the exercise I'm doing today.

    Curves closing was really a blessing in disguise for me. Why are Curves and other gyms/fitness facilities always in a strip mall with food franchises? I belonged to three Curves. One next to Subway, one next to Pat's Pizzeria and the last one next to Alicia's - a Mexican bakery. The Vasa I go to sometimes has a Little Caesar's, Nepali Chulo Indian restaurant and several other eateries in the parking lot. One of the places I do Zumba has Mexican food and ice cream right next door. All of it smells incredible after a workout and very tempting. My last Curves started having an instructor come in and teach Zumba. I had never heard of Zumba before, but tried it and loved it right away. I was terrible at it for about four months, but refused to give up and eventually started to learn the steps and moves. Dancing as exercise is a great concept, especially if you love music which I absolutely do. Many years ago before I started my journey I took some country line dancing classes and loved that also. My mom to this day goes country line dancing multiple days every week and she loves it.

While I was still at Curves, one of the younger ladies there told me about a gym she belonged to nearby that had an awesome Zumba instructor and encouraged me to go with her and try it. So I did and she was right! The instructor was incredible. She had so much energy, excellent music and choreography. It was $5 for a one hour class or $25 for a monthly membership. At first I just paid $5 per class, but when I started going to multiple classes per week I decided to get a membership at JVA (Jordan Valley Athletic Club). When Curves owner Claudette announced that at the end of March seven years ago they would be closing permanently, I was sad and nervous, but it forced me to embrace change, step outside my comfort zone and recognize I was not challenging myself with fitness. I had outgrown and progressed past what Curves had to offer, but I didn't push myself or look for anything else until I had no choice.

Once Curves closed, I kept doing Zumba, but also started trying out other classes at JVA to replace the strength training I thought I was getting at Curves. I tried spinning, kickboxing, pilates, HIIT (high intensity interval training), tabata, boot camp, weight lifting and TBC (total body conditioning). I settled into a new routine of boot camp, TBC, weight lifting and Zumba taking up to a maximum of 9 classes a week. I usually didn't take any classes on Friday nights and the gym was closed on Sundays. I would go to kickboxing or Zumba on Saturday mornings if we were not off somewhere hiking.

When I first started my Curves replacement classes at JVA, I was nervous. I didn't know what to expect. The class instructors were great, but at first I struggled to learn and keep up with what we were doing in each class. And oh how I suffered at first! My body was really getting challenged more than it had ever been. Muscles I had probably never used before were getting used. After some of these classes, I would be so sore for days. Getting on and off of the toilet alone was an unpleasant event. I didn't want to stop taking the classes because I knew the strength training and things I was learning and muscles I was using were good for me, but I had to do something to alleviate the soreness.

    I had noticed this guy for several weeks in the back of some of the classes. He would be lifting these huge hand weights (35 pounds each I believe) and it seemed effortless like it was nothing while I was suffering after using five pound hand weights or less. He had huge muscular arms. I decided to approach this guy and ask for his help or suggestions. I've never been a shy person and I'm direct so I just walked up to him after a class one day and said hi, I need your help. The way he looked at me was like why is this white woman talking to me and what does she want? I've also learned in Utah (unlike Delaware where I'm from) that English is not everyone's first language. Maybe he didn't understand my words or my accent?

    After we kind of got past that, he did offer suggestions most of which I implemented immediately. I started taking magnesium every day (I still do). I started taking amino acids and drinking a protein shake after all classes except Zumba. And boy did it help immensely! I kept taking all of these classes until JVA was sold to a new owner several years ago. It was really sad when they closed. It was a small gym with some incredible instructors and some amazing members. It had more of a family feel to it and you got to know the regular members and see them in the classes you took as well as the people that worked at the front desk. I feel like I made some friendships there and I don't get to see most of those people anymore, but I still think of them often.

    While I was still going to JVA, the lady that suggested I go there and try the Zumba and I trained for and completed a 5K run. Running is not my specialty, but I enjoyed training for and completing a 5K run and I do still run on occasion when the weather is good (has to be at least 50 degrees with no precipitation) and I feel like I am lacking or needing some additional exercise. Whenever I do, it's usually on Sundays in the park connected to my development. Before training for the 5K, she and I went to the Salt Lake Running Company. They videoed us running on a treadmill for about 30 seconds, measured our feet and brought out running shoes they recommended in different brands. It was an awesome experience, and investment. I ended up with a pair of hot pink neutral ride Nike pegasus sneakers. The first time I put those Nikes on my feet, I thought I was walking on a cloud. Did I mention I have flat feet? My son recently decided he wanted to start running, so I took him to Salt Lake Running too! He also has flat feet.

When JVA closed suddenly (I think we got 2 weeks or less notice) I didn't know what I was going to do. I didn't want to lapse with my exercise routine so I had to come up with a plan. Several of the JVA instructors were also teaching classes at Vasa which is more of a mainstream traditional chain gym. A lot of the instructors taught classes really early in the morning at Vasa (5:30 am) and while I am an early morning person, I'm not an early morning workout person. I'm more of a 9-10 am workout person if I'm gonna go in the morning, but I start work at 5:30 or 6 am so that is out unless it's Saturday or I have a day off. The JVA setup was perfect. All classes and any equipment needed for those classes were in the same big room. I decided to join Vasa and get the membership that allowed you to go to any Vasa location. I also started going to different Herbalife locations following Zumba instructors I like. I was not really and to this day still not enjoying traveling around to different Vasa and Herbalife locations trying to get my classes in or trying to put a schedule together each week of where I needed to be and when, but I did my best to keep my fitness routine in place. Unfortunately I got down to one weight lifting class per week and 3-4 Zumba classes due to times of classes and locations. I still really miss the convenience of JVA.

All my life or at least since I was seventeen, I've been on an emotional seesaw or rollercoaster with my body image. When I was a senior in high school. I thought I was fat (I was about 140 pounds) so I put myself on a starvation diet, started taking Dexatrim (I wonder if it still exists?) and refused to wear shorts because I didn't want anyone to see my legs. Wow, was I ridiculous! For the past 30 years, I've gone back and forth. When I was fat, I wore shorts all the time, but most of them were long and I bought my clothes extra

Keep It Off

big thinking I was hiding my body. As I'm writing this, it sounds so stupid to me! As I started my weight loss and fitness journey, the thing I've hated the most is my legs. They seriously look like cottage cheese and the more weight I lose the worse I think they look.

Some years I've been like, I've lost a lot of weight and I'm wearing those cute shorts, I don't care what anyone thinks! The past couple of years I've been like eww my legs are so gross I'm only wearing Bermuda shorts in public. I even bought a new bathing suit with Bermuda shorts. I've seen a plastic surgeon about getting some work done primarily on my upper legs/thighs, but I haven't moved forward. I don't know what the right answer is here. I know there is no easy miracle cure that is legit or any of these miracle products either. I've tried every face cream known to man (I don't see any difference). Recently every night I was putting this Get Dreamy cream on my legs thinking if I keep using it, I'm suddenly going to have these amazing looking legs? Have I mentioned that I have the biggest knees I've ever seen on a woman my size? Why when some people lose weight everything goes back in place and they look so good and for others like me everything is a saggy mess? How do some of these ladies that have 3 kids and lost weight not have a single stretch mark? Why don't I love my body as it is? Why do I care what other people will think if I wear shorts?

What does success look like to you? How do you know if you've achieved success? I've lost almost 100 pounds, maintained the weight loss for over a decade, improved my diet, exercise and made moving my body part of my daily routine. I don't know if I would say I'm fully successful and I may never be. Maybe I'm okay with that? I've definitely reached or exceeded many goals, but each time I do, I re-evaluate and set new goals. Maybe I haven't reached satisfaction with my body yet. Maybe I never will?

We are way harder on ourselves than others are. Some people will say you look great! Why don't I just say thank you and accept it? Instead my response is usually something like are you kidding have you seen these jiggly flabby legs yuck. Or my friend will say look at those muscles (on my arms) and I respond with what muscles? Have you seen these bat wings? I think I will always be a work in progress.

Keep It Off

There are so many things I don't like about my body it's easier to list the things I do like because the list is so short: I think my feet are cute, I like the color of my eyes–kind of somewhere between green, blue and gray. I like how my shoulders look in a tank top. Maybe my calves. That was really hard! I really had to think about it and I didn't even come up with five things. I really need to come up with a fifth thing that I like about my body.

That is seriously sad because the list of things I don't like is really long: I don't like my cottage cheese upper legs and thighs, my jiggly saggy pockmarked butt, my gigantic knees, the stretch marks on my stomach, back and legs, my bat wing arms. I don't like the mole or whatever it is under my nose that grows dark hairs, the wrinkles around my eyes, the hairs that grow on my chin. I don't like the dark spots on my face. I don't like my super old looking hands.

Okay, maybe the lists of likes and dislikes are pretty even. I was able to think of some more likes: I like my wrists, A-cup boobs, nose and lips. I'm kind of proud of my stomach considering the amount of weight I lost. It's not totally flat but doesn't look bad and you can see some ab definition. I have a love/hate relationship with my wild, unique, naturally curly hair that I sometimes straighten as long as I'm not in humidity or rain. I'm kind of neutral on my neck. If you can love all of your body as it is right now, that's awesome. I may never get there, but I will never stop working on it.

Grilled Chicken & Diet Pepsi

It's Your Journey. No One Else's

I've never been a competitive person and this journey is not a competition or a team sport. I hate to be selfish, but this journey is about me. Nobody else. I will succeed or fail with support and love or insecurity and jealousy.

I apply this kind of thinking to all of the roles I play in life - wife, mom, sister, daughter, aunt, friend and employee. I like to be my best self in all of these roles. In order to do so I first have to take care of myself. This is something I have to continuously remind myself of, because my natural tendency is to put my needs aside and take care of everyone else. You have to figure out what taking care of yourself looks like and then do it. One of the ways I take care of myself is working a half day on Fridays as often as I possibly can and taking the other half off just for me to do whatever I want.

I did this last Friday and my afternoon looked like this: I went to a Zumba class, came home and showered, made myself some lunch and sat on the front porch to eat, went for a walk in my neighborhood while listening to music, read my latest mystery book in my lounge chair on the patio for about two hours while sipping a massive Diet Pepsi. It was six hours of doing the things that help me destress, relax, refresh, and regroup, so that I could be effective when I started back to wearing all my different hats.

Another way I take care of myself is going with my friend to get a pedicure every five to six weeks. Worth every penny! Best money I spend! Sitting in a massage chair with your feet in hot water, massage on your legs and feet, hot wax, hot towel, and getting your toes painted while talking to your friend. It doesn't get much better! So I ask you, what does taking care of yourself look like? If you can't remember the last time you did any self-care, today is the best day to start.

Keep It Off

Is There Such a Thing as Dressing Inappropriately for Your Size?

Yes, I believe there is. I may not be popular in saying this, but I feel compelled to talk about it so I will apologize in advance to those I offend. Also, let me say this: although I struggle with body image, I'm all about loving yourself and your body. Everyone should love themselves right now, and that means you love your body, too! What I don't understand (and never have) is wearing clothing that exposes a lot of skin in public. This goes for anyone, but it's especially true when you are extremely obese and/or don't have the body for it. Maybe go for it in the privacy of your own home, but not in public. Nobody wants to see it.

It's really popular right now to wear tight crop tops regardless of size. Seriously, they're really just long bras. I see lots of ladies wearing them from a size zero to the largest possible. I see it at the gym, out shopping, in restaurants. Not to state the obvious, but if it's winter/cold outside and you have to wear a jacket/coat, you should also probably wear a shirt and not just a bra! I used to see it at the beach all the time– ladies in bikinis that designers shouldn't even make in those sizes. I've often wondered if these people actually looked in the mirror and said, "Damn, I look good!" before they went out. Are family and friends no longer willing to honestly help you out, to be honest with you and say hey that outfit really isn't flattering on you? If so, that is really sad. I know my BFF has always had my back on this topic, and if needed she has been brutally honest with me. I sincerely appreciate it.

Here's a typical conversation in the dressing room at Kohl's:

Me: How about this shirt?

BFF: Um, no Charlie Brown!

Me: How about this shirt?

BFF: Does every shirt you buy have to have stripes on it?

LOL

The Scale is Not Always a Friend
Let's talk about fluctuations in weight. They say you shouldn't weigh yourself every day, but I do, often multiple times a day. I only count my morning naked daily weigh-in and my monthly Weight Watchers

weigh-in (obviously not naked). I've been doing this for so many years. What I've learned is you can expect weight and scale fluctuations. They may not always make sense, but they can be very motivating. I use my monthly Weight Watchers weigh-ins to calibrate my home scale. Most of the time the Weight Watchers scale is half a pound higher than my home scale, but so far no more than one pound higher. I'm all about the scale. When it goes down, I'm like, "Yeah!" Fist pump! When it goes up, I'm like, "Damn it!" So I'm either happy and motivated or pissed and motivated.

Then there are times when I can eat pizza and ice cream and the scale goes down the next day or even the next couple of days. Other times I think I'm being super good with food choices and accurate with portion sizes but the scale goes up. Those are the days I want to throw the scale across the room or out the window.

Weight can fluctuate for many reasons—hormones, water retention, salt intake, to name a few—but if you are in it for the long haul, just use the scale as a tool to monitor your results. Unless over a period of time (you have to figure out what period of time you are comfortable with) you are trending in the wrong direction, do not worry too much about day to day weight fluctuations. This is kind of off topic, but every month when I go to the Weight Watchers in Murray, Utah for my weigh-in, I see a poster in the window that says something like: How would you measure success if the scale didn't exist? I think about that every month and my answer is I don't know. Would I base it on how my clothes fit? If my clothes feel loose, my weight is going down. If my clothes feel tight, my weight is going up. Would I base it on how I feel such as energy level? How else could you measure success on a weight loss and fitness journey? Maybe measure specific body parts on a monthly basis? The scale is how I measure.

Random Thoughts

When I was a size 16 plus, they had special separate stores for those sizes (20+ years ago). You really couldn't find much in those sizes at any regular stores. So, my BFF and I did most of our shopping at Lane Bryant. At the time both of us were about a size 18 and we are both about 5 feet 1 inch tall. I often wondered where the Amazon women were that they made the clothes for. I would try on pants and would be walking on them or have to make a triple cuff. No thanks. I would try on long sleeve shirts and they would come down past my fingers or again do the triple cuff. Again no thanks. Summer clothes worked though - the shorts came down past my knees and the shirts hung down past my butt with sleeves almost to the elbow. The shirts looked like tents. And what was I doing wearing leggings at that size? Wow. Anyway, just because people are fat doesn't mean they are tall or long.

Random thought: I've never been fat enough to have to buy two seats on an airplane. I wonder what that feels like.

I can't sleep without melatonin and half a Kirkland sleep aid. It's been like this for about 10 years. My mind will just not shut off/down. I just automatically take both about 30 minutes before I want to go to sleep otherwise I'm just tossing and turning and thinking for hours. I hate that I have become dependent on these. I've tried to talk to the doctor about it and he just said to take Benadryl at night. Insert eye roll. Benadryl does knock me out, but it leaves me groggy the next day. My method doesn't make me groggy.

As sleep may be a key component of weight loss, I would like to figure this out. Also, melatonin gives me weird dreams. I recently had a dream that the police were searching my house. I asked how much longer they were going to be because they said 20 minutes and it had already been 2 hours. Then I looked at the clock and thought to myself they better hurry up because I have Zumba in an hour. Then the alarm woke me up.

Well, I gained about four pounds in four weeks after my neck surgery. The first week my friend flew in to help me and we were not eating very healthy or doing any exercise other than a little walking. The second and third weeks I tried to be a lot better with my diet and walk more. The second week, I didn't work, but the third week I did. The fourth week people from work flew in for our quarterly business meeting. I went into the office for three days and went out to dinner for two nights. My diet was mostly out the window those days, but I did try to walk as much as I could. I sure did overeat a couple days. All in all, I'm

Keep It Off

happy with the four pounds. I went for my post surgery follow up Thursday afternoon. They took x-rays, removed the bandage, said everything looked and sounded great. I was cleared to slowly start doing Zumba again! I didn't like how my neck looked once the bandage was off, but I hoped it would get better over time. I went to my first Zumba class in over a month on Saturday. It felt so good to be back! My diet was back on track and I had already lost two of the four pounds I gained. Just a short detour on my journey. By Monday, I had just finished my second Zumba class post surgery. I felt amazing! Lots of energy, great mood. Zumba is so many things to me as I've mentioned ad nauseam, I'm sure. Zumba is like therapy to me in addition to all the other things. I missed all of it so much. I'm taking it slow, but so glad to be back! I've already lost 3.5 of the four pounds I gained. I'm sure I can get rid of the remaining half pound in no time. I've always had a lot of energy, but wow I'm bursting with it now! Look out!

Getting past consumption is tough. Everywhere you look you see ads, posters, coupons, commercials, food trucks, fast food restaurants, Girl Scout cookies.

Everything looks good, sounds good, there is availability everywhere. The power of suggestion. Convenience stores. 90% of the brain responds to images, feelings, experiences, while only 10% of the brain is logical which makes a weight loss and fitness journey so challenging. You have to know yourself, find your will power, self control, find ways to manage your consumption. Facebook is full of ads, but it hasn't impacted me with food and drinks yet. It has caused me to shop at several places online and want things, but we're not talking about shopping right now. I don't really watch television, but others at my house do and sometimes I'm in the room reading and I'll see an ad for food and boy do I want it sometimes. Or at least I want to try it while secretly hoping equal parts it tastes great or I don't like it. Or I can have just a little to get the desire out of my system.

> I'm sorry for what I said when I was hungry.

The other day I went to Crumbl (cookies) to get my friend a thank you gift card because she tried them when she was here, liked them and they just opened

Keep It Off

one near her. I told myself I was not buying any cookies as tempting as they are. The clerk gave me a free brookie cookie - half brownie and half chocolate chip and dang it, I ate it! Last week at a work event they had Red Iguana catered in. I ate two chicken enchiladas. They were so delicious. The mole was amazing. I can't stop thinking about those enchiladas! Yesterday I got in my mind that I wanted Oreo ice cream and a hot soft pretzel? All of these things come from past experiences. I didn't get any of these things. Just say no!

Keep Saying No to the Oreos

No Excuses with Exercise

If you're really serious about keeping weight off, you have to have a goal and a plan—and you have to stick to it. Excuses show up fast, and I've learned the hard way that without structure, it's too easy to fall off track. That's why I always have a plan, and I've learned what does and doesn't work for me.

Some people thrive working out at home, but not me. I've tried it countless times. The minute I try to exercise at home, I remember something I "need" to do—laundry, dishes, calling a friend. It's too easy to get distracted. For me, exercise has to happen outside my house. It has to be an intentional outing, a place I go, a class I attend. Once I'm in that setting, I commit. And it's not just about the workout—it's the people too. That social connection makes a big difference.

Over the years, I've been part of a lot of gyms and classes. I started with Curves, just half a mile from my house. It was easy, familiar, and full of wonderful women I loved seeing. When I moved to Utah, one of the first things I did was transfer my membership. At one point, Curves offered Zumba classes for a few extra dollars. They weren't consistent, but they introduced me to a whole new kind of workout that I instantly loved.

A friend told me about a Zumba class at Jordan Valley Athletic Club (JVA), and I decided to try it. It was only $5 per class and quickly became a new favorite. I was still going to Curves too, so for a while I had two memberships—one for strength training, one for Zumba. Some might see that as excessive, but it worked for me. That $60 a month investment in my health was worth far more than spending that money on fast food or new clothes I didn't need.

Eventually, Curves closed, and I transitioned fully to JVA. It was farther from home—five miles instead of half a mile—but I adjusted. I missed the convenience and the familiar faces, but I met new people and found a similar sense of community. Then JVA was sold and shut down, which threw me into another round of adjustment.

I followed some of my favorite instructors to other places—Vasa, local recreation centers, and Herbalife locations offering Zumba. I joined Vasa for $20 a month, which gave me access to any location in any state. It seemed like a good deal, but they didn't offer many of the classes I wanted without upgrading to a more expensive membership. Meanwhile, I was paying $3-$5 per class at other places. Some weeks I was attending multiple classes per day at different locations. It took planning and flexibility, but I made it work.

Then COVID hit, and everything shut down. Like so many people, I scrambled to figure out what to do. I even hunted down outdoor Zumba classes and drove over 20 miles just to find one. And just when I felt like I was finding a rhythm again, my family and I got COVID—twice. We were lucky to have mild cases, but it was still a setback. It would have been so easy to quit, but I knew quitting would only make me feel worse.

When things reopened, I tried to get back to my old schedule. But the changes kept coming. Some instructors I loved weren't teaching anymore. Vasa no

Keep It Off

longer offered the classes I liked. Some Herbalife locations started requiring product purchases—$10 to $13 just to attend a class. It wasn't sustainable. I started skipping classes I normally loved. Not because I didn't want to go, but because I couldn't justify the expense.

Even with all these challenges, I've stayed committed to exercise. Right now, I'm doing Zumba four to six days a week. I've found new instructors and locations. I've adapted again, because I know how important it is to keep going. Zumba brings me joy. It clears my head. It relieves my stress. It keeps me grounded.

> Doing what you love never goes out of style.

That's what a plan does. It gives you something to come back to. Something that keeps you anchored.

A plan helps you decide instead of delay. It helps you pivot instead of panic. It makes the hard times manageable.

Now I'm facing another obstacle: two severely pinched nerves in my neck. The pain in my left arm and shoulder has been intense. I'm scheduled for surgery in less than six weeks. One of the first things I asked the surgeon was, "When can I get back to Zumba?" That's how important it is to me.

I'm already working on a modified recovery plan. I'll do what I can during recovery, something gentle but consistent. I won't give myself permission to fall apart. I've come too far. I could easily use surgery as an excuse to give up—curl up on the couch, watch TV, eat ice cream out of the carton—but I won't. I've worked too hard for that.

Exercise isn't about perfection. It's about persistence. It's about making it work in the middle of life's messes. It's about knowing yourself and finding what makes you feel strong, confident, and capable. You don't have to love the same routines I do. You just have to find what works for you—and keep doing it.

Keep showing up. Keep saying no to the Oreos. And when life throws you curveballs—and it will—adjust your plan, but never give up on yourself.

Endless Highway

The Big Move

I told you how over sixteen years ago, I moved from Delaware to Utah. The Discover site I was working at was closing as our primary purpose was processing payments, and many customers were paying online. Discover decided it was no longer cost-effective to have two locations for Payment Processing.

It wasn't an easy decision to make. I had lived my entire life up to 38 years old in Delaware near all of my family. This was in 2008 when the housing market crashed. Many businesses were closing locally and gas prices were sky high—about the same as they are now. I was a 38-year-old woman with no college education, a 7-year-old son, and 20 years of service at Discover Financial Services. My options were to take a severance package and try to find a decent paying job in a terrible job market and a lot of people to compete with or stay with Discover and accept an opportunity in Utah, moving across the country.

Although it was a hard decision to make, I think I've grown as a person and learned so much as a result. The move forced me to meet new people at work and outside of work. I had to learn how to find my way around a new place. Delaware only had one major freeway. I had to make new friends and develop good relationships with new business associates.

It was even a challenge to figure out where I wanted to go grocery shopping, buy appliances and furniture, get good child care, find a doctor, dentist, and the best takeout. I had to figure out where the hospital was, the school, the gym, and where to rent a house. Hardest of all, we had to decide what to do on weekends now that we were 2400 miles away from all our family and friends.

I do still miss my family and my BFF of over 40 years (and other friends and business associates). I miss them especially on holidays, birthdays, and other fun family events and when anyone is not well or in the hospital and I can't be there with them.

But I've learned to love the outdoors—national parks, hiking, waterfalls, walking in local parks, reading on the patio. We take day trips all over the place. I've met people from Mexico, Venezuela, Argentina, Ecuador, Peru, and many other Latin countries. I've worked with people from India, learned about all of their cultures, festivals, and food.

Once I was no longer able to attend any family events and started doing physical things for fun such as hiking, I lost 20 pounds in just a few short months. I went from 145 to 125 just like that!

I also started paying more attention to the amount of food I ate and the type of food I ate. Gone were the piles of macaroni and cheese at every family event, the chocolate eclair cake, and many other things. These became treats I only made when going to friends' houses or events which were much less frequent than when I lived in Delaware and had so many events with friends and family.

Also, when we did have family events, the variety and quantities were limitless—like a huge buffet with usually at least 30 people as each person would bring something to the events. Now in Utah, we only have one main dish, a couple side dishes, bread/rolls, and one dessert instead of tons. It took my guys some getting used to, but here we are 16 years later.

Before moving to Utah, I had never eaten food from or the following cuisines: Indian, Thai, Colombian, real Mexican. I had never been to stores they would shop at. Now they are some of my favorite places to shop and eat.

I go to Perez Market for carne asada and Anaya's for chorizo and chicken, La Selecta for chicharron, and many other things. There's Panaderia Alicia's for sweet bread. And then there's La Casa del Tamal, El Cabrito for the best enchiladas in Utah, Nepali Chulo, fresh carnitas, tacos, tamales, arepas, naan, chicken tikka masala, yellow curry, chicken vindaloo. The list could go on and on.

I got an awesome analogy today from a very wise woman (Lara) and a tagline that is perfect—"Don't Let Go of the Wheel." A weight loss and fitness journey really is like going on a road trip/journey and driving to get to your destination, except you realize once you get there that the journey never ends. To keep the weight off, you have to maintain the same disciplines you developed while you were losing the weight.

Keep It Off

Few people drive straight through without stopping. Most people make several stops along the way. As you drive towards your destination, you may stop to get gas and use the restroom. You may stop to stretch your legs and get something to eat. All regular stops on a road trip.

But there are many other mostly unplanned stops along the way that could happen, delaying your arrival at your final destination. You could make a wrong turn and have to find your way back to your path. You may get lost and not realize it for a period of time and have to backtrack. You may have to take a detour that takes you hours and/or several miles out of your way. You could run into road construction causing a long delay in your trip. You could hit a pothole and get a flat tire. If you have a jack and a spare, great! If you don't, you may have to wait for roadside assistance or a tow truck. You could need some other type of unplanned maintenance on your vehicle causing unexpected delays.

When you head out on a road trip, you may attempt to prepare for unforeseen circumstances, but you can't anticipate all obstacles you may encounter along the way. On a weight loss and fitness journey, you may also encounter planned and unplanned stops, detours, and other delays—and that's okay. How long it takes to get to your final destination is up to you!

Caravaning Makes the Journey More Fun
There will be days that are tougher than others. Recently, I was thinking about my disappointment with being up 3–5 pounds, how my stomach looked bloated, I was still overeating pita chips, and my Diet Pepsi intake had reached an all-time high. I felt out of control.

Even if there were reasons why I am or may be experiencing some of these things, there were also definitely improvements I could make to reel it in big time. I was thinking I needed to go back to my old rule from years ago where I only allowed myself one glass of Diet Pepsi for lunch and one for dinner. Trust me, this was a huge improvement/reduction for me. I also needed to stop with the extra pita chips. Just make myself stop. This Diet Pepsi and pita chips thing was a huge change for me. If I wanted to be successful, I needed to get mentally prepared. For me, getting mentally prepared looks like self-talk and sounds something like this: "Girl, you have worked so hard, you have come so far, you've been here before and you can do this! You've built a solid foundation and set up the structure to succeed. Time and again you have made promises to yourself, set goals and surpassed them. You can do anything you put your mind to! You've got this!" At this point, though, I didn't know how I was going to motivate myself to achieve these goals.

Then one night I went to my regular 7 p.m. Zumba class and found out they were having a 21-day Fitness Challenge! I love when things happen like this! This may be exactly the extra motivation or nudge I need to deal with some of my current issues and see what I can do in 21 days!

All I had to do was get weighed, measured, and pay $25. I didn't exactly understand the rules to win, but that's okay (all the information was in Spanish). Winning would be a bonus. I was using this as a way to improve myself and cut some bad habits. I was also striving for my ultimate goal of weighing 105 pounds, which would put me at exactly 100 pounds lost. All of my previous efforts seemed to push this goal further away than closer to it.

I decided to make a list of goals or things I wanted to focus on for 21 days to see how I did. I came up with five of my own goals for the challenge:

1. **Significantly reduced diet soda intake.** I allowed myself one can at lunch and one can at dinner at least Monday through Friday. It might not have seemed like a huge improvement, but trust me—it was. I had been drinking up to two 2-liters daily before starting the challenge.
2. **Stopped overeating pita chips.** I counted out my portion and didn't go get the bag for overindulgence afterward. If I wanted more, I counted out another portion. I stuck to no more than two portions at a time.
3. **Drank more water.** Since I was drinking less Diet Pepsi, I had to have something because I was a very thirsty girl. I had previously been drinking 64 ounces of water per day.
4. **Ate healthier meals and snacks.** More chicken, less pork. More protein, fewer carbohydrates. I would have liked to say more

fruit and vegetables, but that has always been a hard one for me. I might have to be rewired or hypnotized to fix that. No more pork rinds! I did some research and ended up with low-sugar granola, dark chocolate Dove individuals, and cashews for snacks. I tried to avoid eating between meals unless I got really hungry and couldn't make it to the next meal.
5. **Worked towards the ultimate goal of 105 pounds.** Wouldn't it have been cool to say I had lost 100 pounds?! I thought so.

I was six days in and it was going okay. Goals 1–4 were on track. There was a group of seven of us in the challenge and Ana had started a group chat for us. It was fun posting pictures of our meals and encouraging each other in the chat.

Group motivation isn't usually my thing, but I was really enjoying it. It was nice to see the ladies when we were at Zumba also. It was also cool to try some of the Herbalife products (part of the challenge was to buy three products per week).

Since I was the only one not fluent in Spanish, it was kind of interesting. I had no idea what to order. LOL. This week I had a chocolate protein shake, a cookies-and-cream protein shake, and some type of berry energy drink. All were good and I think I might have drunk a strawberry!

Goal 5 was not going great so far. I would be lying if I said I wasn't disappointed. I started the challenge at 110.6 and I was only down to 109.0. I felt like I was killing it and should see more results on the scale. But that was okay. I was persistent, dedicated, motivated, and determined. I would just keep going and see what happens. There were still 15 days to go.

> **Results happen over time, not overnight. Work hard, stay consistent, and be patient.**

I did well with goals 1–4 all the way through, but I continued to struggle with goal 5. During the second week, I managed to get the scale down to 106.4 one day, but by Monday, I was right back to 110.5. That meant I had lost just one pound in two weeks.

Keep It Off

Really? Seriously? I was giving it everything I had. I had even significantly reduced weekend desserts! I felt disappointed with the results on the scale but really good about everything else. Significantly cutting back on Diet Pepsi had reduced my bloating a lot. Holding myself more accountable to my portions and Weight Watchers points felt good, and I didn't feel hungry or deprived. One week to go—I wanted to see what I could do. I had also stopped putting flavored syrup in my Diet Pepsi during the challenge.

By the end of the 21-day challenge, I had lost five pounds and achieved all my other goals! I didn't win, but I still felt like a winner. I had even lost an inch around my waist and got closer to my ultimate goal than I had ever been—and the lowest I had ever weighed: 105.4, even if it was just for two days! And the best part was that it was fun. I planned to continue even though the challenge was over and to keep trying to reach my ultimate goal. It was attainable and within my reach. I considered taking a small break on Thanksgiving Day to eat a bowl of ice cream or a cookie, but then I'd get right back to it.

I learned so many things during the 21 day challenge. No order, but here they are:

1. The Herbalife horchata is delicious and nutritious. I'm going to say it helped with all my goals during the challenge so I can justify continuing to get it whether it's true or not! LOL.
2. I started eating a smaller breakfast and most days that worked perfectly. On the few days I got hungry before lunch, I would have a low fat protein shake or one of my healthier snacks.
3. I learned I really don't like dark chocolate and I'm not really an in between meals snacker. I prefer a smaller breakfast and bigger lunch and dinner.
4. I said I had 5 goals, but I ended up with more just going through the process. The 2 extra goals were: eat healthier on the weekends with meals and significantly reducing dessert intake on weekends.
5. I didn't miss Diet Pepsi or desserts as much as I thought I would. I was able to reduce my portions and still be satisfied and not hungry.

6. I was perfectly happy with healthier and cleaner food for Friday take out night such as a half chicken Caesar salad from Panera or a chicken bowl from Zao. I was satisfied with a piece of Dove milk chocolate for a dessert instead of a huge bowl of ice cream, a big Crumbl cookie or sweet bread from the Mexican bakery.
7. I also think it was a good experience for my family. We usually rotate Friday night take out, but during the challenge we didn't. I think they learned healthier takeout is still yummy and there are other choices besides burgers and pizza.

Just a few weeks after the challenge ended, my hard work paid off. It took me 20 years, but finally on 12/2/23 I reached my ultimate goal for at least one day for the first time ever! When I started my journey I weighed 205 pounds and when I got on the scale on 12/2/23, I weighed 104.5! I can officially say I've lost 100 pounds! I was so excited and couldn't believe it. I even took a picture while standing on the scale! Now that I am here, this is where I would like to stay. For the first time in my entire adult life, I don't need to lose any weight! I can truly and completely be in maintenance mode! I worked so hard to get here, but it was worth it. I've never felt better! And I want to share all of it to help others.

The Destination is the Journey: Enjoy It!
When I'm exercising, primarily doing Zumba 4–6 days a week for an hour, I tell myself I'm a badass, I'm killing it, I've got this! I'm 55 years old, jumping around and working out like I'm 20 or something. I'm motivated and energized. I don't really know if I'm a badass or if I'm killing it, but in my mind I am and that's all that matters.

Of course, there are also times when I'm saying things in my head like oh my God I'm going to die, this class is killing me, why is it so hot in here—but only for a couple minutes so that's okay. LOL.

I can't get enough Zumba and that's good because I need exercise and I enjoy it so much. It's not a chore or something I dread doing. I actually love it and can't wait to get there. I'm always looking for a new class or instructor so I can get to at least four classes a week. I'm loyal to my usual places and will continue to be, but sometimes classes get canceled because we don't have enough people to make the class worthwhile/at least break even to pay the instructor, or they close for holidays when bigger places/gyms are open. I try to always have a backup plan.

I often follow instructors I really like to other locations and I meet new instructors that I end up liking and follow them too.

> My drug of choice –Zumba Fitness.

Zumba works for me for so many reasons: I'm social, I like to learn about different cultures, and I love music. I've been a music lover my entire life across many genres. Every class is like a dance party. The music has great rhythm and beats. I have favorites at each class or with each instructor. Some of the moves are basic aerobics like jumping jacks, but some are different in many ways.

Some are regular moves like salsa or cumbia. Some are more exotic or difficult and even after many years practicing my body still won't move like that. I have an app on my phone called Sound Hound and when there are songs in class that I like, I activate Sound Hound so I can get the name of the song and the artist.

Later I will buy the songs and add them to my Zumba playlist on my phone. Then I listen to it in the car, walking or running in the park, when I'm in the shower.

Each instructor has a different style. Sometimes instructors have the same music with different moves, but most instructors have songs that others don't. I keep adding to my Zumba playlist and the songs remind me of instructors past and present.

I truly miss instructors that move on or decide to stop teaching. If they come back, I will be at their classes! My current active favorites whose classes I take regularly are: Arcy Leon Corona, Erika Leon, Julia Leon (at Arcy's or Erika's classes), Diana Munoz Coronado, and Beto Montero Rodal. If I can catch a class with Rocio Diaz or Irvin Juarez I'm there!

Recently my buddy Christopher Santana got certified and I just tried his class last night. It was great and he's an awesome guy! Last week I tried a class given by one of the owners of Ole Nutrition—Eva Galvan. Wow. I love her energy, her smile, and her class was great!

Sometimes you have to get past or overlook your issues to be successful. I love Zumba so much and I give it everything I've got in every class. I am always sweating and overheating. This is because of how hard I work in the class, menopause, and having cholinergic urticaria (an increase in body temperature often causing hives).

I do not let any of these things stop me and I truly enjoy every class.

Cheese Fries & Samosas

Another Blessing in Disguise

When COVID hit, gyms closed and some instructors moved on to other things never to return. Once again I was challenged to find ways to creatively keep my fitness routine going. As I stated earlier, at the beginning of my journey I wasn't good at getting to the gym after going home first. When COVID hit, I had already been working from home full time for about two years so going to a class at night was my primary social interaction. I've always treated my exercise classes as another appointment, meeting or commitment on my daily calendar to keep me accountable, not get wrapped up in other things at home or make excuses for not going or not doing it. This time I really didn't have a choice and I wanted to keep going. I had this six week Kettlebell DVD program that I had done years ago and I dusted that off and did the whole thing again except this time I would do 2-3 workouts at a time instead of just one to try to equal one 60 minute class. I started running in the park multiple days a week to offset or equal my missed Zumba classes, I also started walking more. I would reach out to anyone I knew asking about any open gyms or Zumba classes anywhere and I would go to any class anywhere with any instructor that I could find.

I've never understood why people don't go to a class if there is a substitute or new instructor. Every instructor you've ever had was new to you at some point. I've found some awesome instructors that I love trying substitutes, new locations or new instructors when instructors decide to move on to other things in their lives. My fitness routine does not stop because a gym closes, an instructor leaves or a pandemic hits. Since COVID stabilized, I have pretty much only been doing Zumba Monday to Thursday at 7 pm at Herbalife locations with whoever the instructor is (sometimes me). Some truly awesome instructors continue to come and go and people attending the classes come and go too, but I just keep hanging on. I still have my Vasa membership and will go there for a Zumba class if my regular class gets cancelled and I can't find anywhere else to go. I'm disappointed in myself that I haven't continued at least one strength training or weight lifting class per week. I keep saying I'm going to post COVID, but I haven't yet. I'm not sure what is holding me back. I really have no excuse.

Vacations and Business Trips/Breaks in Routine
I do struggle to keep on track with my diet and exercise routines when on vacation or a business trip. I am doing better with it than in the past, but I still have a lot of room for improvement. Maybe it's okay to loosen the reins during these times, but it doesn't have to get out of control. I used to stop tracking food and points while on vacation, but now I track food and points every single day. It's like as soon as I get to the airport or arrive at my temporary location, all of my routines go out the window. I revert back to my old bad overeating habits, making bad food choices and making excuses or ignoring the fact that I am not

> I see you've been eating whatever you want and not exercising – Pants

Keep It Off

exercising. On my most recent business trip to Chicago, I did once again take exercise clothes with me as I usually do and I did go by the hotel gym once, but it was way too crowded. I did continue my step streak while there for five days which is something good. I did have good intentions, but that was all I accomplished.

On the other hand, you should have seen what I ate! I did try to be good at eating 1/2 a chicken Caesar salad at Panera Bread a couple times and I was successful at being good for breakfast since the hotel didn't have it available complementary. I was not good at drinking water. If there was a chips and salsa eating contest, I would have won twice. We also went to my favorite Indian/Pakistani restaurant Sabri Nihari. At one meal I ate pakora, samosa, garlic naan, chicken platter, chicken biryani, tandoori chicken, chicken tikka masala and butter chicken curry. When I go home to Delaware, I am awful! I will for sure be eating Helluva Good sour cream and onion dip with potato chips, buffalo chicken pizza from Pat's, pepperoni pizza and cheese fries from Grotto's, chicken and dumplings at The Smyrna Diner, ice cream cones from

Rita's and polish water ice if I can get it and a cold soft pretzel from Wawa. So delicious, so ridiculous!

As I'm about to land for what I expect to be an incredible once in a lifetime vacation, I'm wondering what I will eat and will I get any exercise in? I have good intentions in mind. I have 9,650 steps for the day already. I ate a sausage, egg and cheese biscuit from Carl's Junior at the airport, no water so far today, Diet Pepsi, two Diet Cokes and some Stacy's naked pita chips on the plane. So I'm on the flight home from the trip. I was able to keep my step streak going by walking my step goal each day, but that was all the exercise I did the whole time. And I over ate every day, but I did track my points every day. I wonder how much weight I gained this time? But it's okay, I'll be back on my exercise routine and eating plan tomorrow or Monday at the latest. Maybe it's okay to take these small breaks from my eating and exercise routines as long as I get back to it as soon as I return from a trip and it's only a few times a year? I know I never want to get back to where I was so that is always front of mind.

Sweet & Spicy

Life Is a Transformational Journey

When I look back over my life, I've really been on a self-transformation journey that started in my early twenties. It's been more than achieving a healthy weight and staying there. As I look back, I can see so many obstacles that I had to overcome. Some of them were downright painful. I could have given up at any one of those turning points, but if I wanted to succeed I had to come up with a solution. So that's what I did.

In every case, those obstacles arose when I took steps to make my life better. Honestly, I think this is true for all of us. Whenever we try to change, things seem to get worse before they get better. You have to face those obstacles if you want to get to that new 'you.' If you can't make it through the obstacles, then you're not going to get there. No pain, no gain. The first things I tried weren't even weight loss, but the same principles applied. I have bad eyesight so in my early twenties I decided to start wearing contacts.

When I first got them, it was a nightmare. There's nothing like poking yourself in the eye every day to raise your stress level–learning how to put them in and take them out, that was the first thing. Then on a trip to Disney World (of course I was on vacation) I had one get stuck behind my eyeball. It was literally on the back of my eyeball, and it took all day to get it out. Then there was a film over that eye that wouldn't go away. So my whole vacation, I couldn't see out of one eye. When I got home, it turned out I had an eye infection. So I had to put in antibiotic eye drops to heal my eye and wait a couple weeks before wearing the contacts again. Crazy stuff. But in the end it was worth it. I had always hated wearing glasses, the glasses never seemed to be clean and I haven't had to wear glasses since except for readers.

A few years later when I was in my early thirties, I decided to get twelve dental crowns replaced–six at a time. Why would I have so many crowns at such a young age, you ask? My teeth have no enamel. My baby teeth were fine, but once they fell out, my permanent teeth came in with no enamel. On top of that, I have a very small mouth (physically anyway–my friends and family would argue it's big and loud and has no off switch). When I was nine years old, I had nine teeth out–some cut out of my gums and some pulled–so there would be enough space in my mouth for the remaining teeth. This was a huge expense for my parents. Then with no enamel, I needed crowns on all the teeth I had left. They didn't have the money for that, so they saved up to have them done one at a time. Doing them one by one had the unfortunate effect of giving me some teeth that were bright white, some that were off-white, and some that were a normal tooth color. None of my teeth were the same color. Talk about embarrassing for a teenager. Everyone always thought or assumed I was in a bad mood because I hated to smile. I didn't want anyone to see my multiple colored teeth and when I did see them in pictures where I did smile I was mortified.

Then when I was 16, my top wisdom teeth were impacted so the top two were pulled and the bottom two were cut out. I swear from the age of five to eighteen, I spent all my time at the dentist. By the time I was 18, I was fed up. I refused to go anymore. Gross I know. When I finally started going back to the dentist, I took the money out of savings and told him if he could do them all at once (not one at a time) I would like to redo all the crowns so they matched–same materials, same color. We compromised with six on the bottom followed by the six on the top. They looked so much better. I was so relieved. I felt so much better about myself. Since then I smile all the time. I've always loved to laugh, and now I can without feeling self-conscious because my teeth look good. Side note, for the past 20+ years I have been going to the dentist regularly like I should. It took a lot of overcoming obstacles to get here, but it was worth it.

Imagine for a second this girl with crazy colored teeth, big thick glasses, and 100 pounds overweight. Add to that my naturally curly hair that had a mind of its own. I was a mess. Another side note: I was happily married with a son then. So it doesn't matter if you look like you want to look to have love and fulfillment. I never did these things to get a man or whatever. It was never for other people. It was for me. I wanted to feel better about how I looked and I wanted to feel better physically and emotionally, and I was willing to do the work that it took to get it done. It was a long journey, and it had a lot of hiccups. And I didn't know if it was going to work. But I pressed on. I hope you will too, in whatever you decide to achieve.

After I got my teeth fixed, I started my weight loss and fitness journey, but I still had a problem–my hair. So my hair came next. I have naturally curly hair and for the first 38 years of my life, I lived in humid and rainy Delaware. During that time my hair had a mind of its own regardless of what I did to it. When I was in junior high, I was bullied by some very mean but very beautiful girls. I won't go into all of that, but what I will say is they said my hair looked like a poodle (they were not wrong). After one specific haircut, they said I looked like Roger Daltrey (again, not wrong). It hurt my feelings, maybe more so because it was true. So when I moved to dry, sunny and much less humid Utah 16 years ago, I got a recommendation to get my hair professionally done at Salon Jace. I got my hair cut, highlighted and straightened, and I love it now. I haven't gone anywhere else since. Jace is a miracle working hair wizard. I have never been good at doing my hair so there were a few rough days and tears until I could figure out how to get as close to Jace's final as possible, but I've got it down now.

Whenever I go somewhere humid or rainy now, or I'm home and feeling lazy, I just put some curly hair products in, scrunch, headband and go. I like it much better straight, but in some climates it doesn't cooperate so why spend the time? Many coworkers or friends in Utah that see my hair curly or natural for the first time ask if I got a perm (I've never had a perm in my entire life) or say they like it that way. Once two male friends at the gym said it looked like a white afro when I returned from a trip to Florida which made me laugh. They must have liked it curly because they would often ask when they would see the white afro again. Not often guys, not often!

Over the years, I have read a lot of books on improving communication skills and how to deal with emotions because I am a very passionate person both when excited and when mad. I am also a very open, direct and outspoken person. This one is an ongoing challenge for me. I continue to work on it; it's always top of mind. It may always be a challenge for me.

Keep It Off

So what comes next in my self-transformation journey? I'm really not sure. One of the goals when I started was to look good (secondary of course to getting healthy). But when you lose half your body weight, what you have left doesn't look like what you imagined. At least it didn't for me. I can say that after losing almost 100 pounds, I do not like how the remaining half looks. I thought I would be happy when I lost weight and got physically fit, but I'm not. Some things come with age and I get that, but the extra skin, the stretch marks, the cottage cheese legs, the bat wings, the over pronounced wrinkles, the jiggly butt. I mean yuck. I don't like how any of it looks and I've worked really hard. Some people say you look great, you are so thin and I think but have you seen me naked? Thank God the answer is no!

> I want to lose weight but I don't want to get caught up in one of those 'eat right and exercise' scams.

So now the argument with myself–should I get the extra skin removed or some other cosmetic things done or just learn to live with what I see in the mirror? Am I really that vain? Do I really want to spend the money? Would I truly be happier? Why don't I love myself as I am, battle scars and all? I have to confess after thinking and talking about it for many years, I did go in January 2023 and talk to someone (I did a lot of research before I made the appointment). I wanted to ask them about what it would take to improve the extra skin on my body.

It wasn't just the extra skin. I have gigantic knees. I guess we all have an area of our bodies that makes us cringe. For me, it's my knees. As a reference, I am five foot one, I weigh 107 pounds and I have to wear an extra large knee brace. Me! In this tiny body. Plus my thighs are like cottage cheese. Yuck. But to be clear, I was not there for any kind of boob job–I'm proud of my A cups.

At the appointment, I wanted to know what it would take and how much it would cost to fix all this. I haven't made a move yet. First, I don't like to spend big money on myself. I'm more of a clearance rack

Under Armour shirts, leggings or sneakers kind of spender. The only time I buy myself full price or expensive things is when I have gift cards or Christmas/birthday money. Second, they told me I would not be able to go to Zumba or exercise for a minimum of two weeks in order to recover properly and I was not feeling that at all.

So will I do it or will I not? Should I or shouldn't I? I told my editor if I really wrote a book, got it published and made enough money to pay for it from the book sales, maybe I would do it. Only time will tell if I can bring myself to do it or not. So I wrote about my self-transformation journey and all the things I've done up to now. My weight loss and fitness, which will be ongoing forever, has been by far the hardest and longest. What I've learned along the way is that you will have to deal with other people's insecurities and it may come unexpectedly and out of nowhere.

Tools for Managing Weight and Setting Goals
Fitness Trackers
I have been walking a lot more the past several years even before COVID. Whoever invented the FitBit is a

genius! I am totally obsessed with that little device! To the point of ridiculousness! I have the FitBit Inspire that clips right to the front of my pants which I prefer (I don't like to wear it like a watch). I have that thing set for the following daily goals: hourly 250 steps for 12 hours a day 7 am to 7 pm, daily steps 12, 650, distance 5 miles, calories burned 1600, active minutes 60. I track my daily progress like a hawk. If I make it to 12,650 steps, I go for 16,650 (equal to 10 Weight Watchers points). If I make it to 16,650 then I go for 20,000 and then 30,000. I think I've hit 40,000 steps a day a few times.

I do everything possible to get my hourly 250 steps goal. I get excited about every badge I earn. I also do everything I can to achieve my daily FitBit goals including going for a streak of consecutive days. As I write this, I'm on day 316 and counting. I've had to start over a few times, but that's okay. I do this by: parking in the back of all parking lots, taking the stairs instead of the elevator, walking during conference calls using a wireless headset, walking while talking to friends and family on the phone, walking instead of sitting while waiting for a flight to board, waiting for a class to start, waiting to get called at an appointment, while reading, going for a walk around the block or in the park when the weather is nice.

Supplements

Until I started taking more intense classes at the gym like boot camp and total body conditioning, I didn't take any dietary supplements. I needed something to help me recover from the soreness. I started with low calorie muscle milk protein shakes for the protein, to help build muscle and post workout recovery. I also started taking amino acids for muscle recovery (it has many other benefits) and magnesium for bone and muscle health and the added benefit of helping keep you regular. Over the years, I've added to my daily supplements to help with various things such as:

- multi vitamins because my diet was lacking in so many things
- fiber therapy, stool softeners, pre & probiotics and bloat relievers to help keep me regular and avoid IBS episodes
- B12 for immune and nervous system health as well as cardiovascular and metabolism support

- biotin to support with hair, skin and nails
- melatonin for sleep support
- folic acid for heart health
- calcium for bone health

For a while, I took collagen which is about the same as biotin. Who knows what I will add next? I guess it depends on what need arises? There are so many different dietary supplements out there. I tend to buy mine from Walmart or Amazon. I don't want to spend a lot of money on supplements although I know a lot of people who do and that's fine if that's what you want. I would rather spend that money on new workout clothes or sneakers! Whether for health reasons or workouts, get the supplements that will help you be the best version of yourself. A lot of men I know that workout, including my son, use creatine which enhances muscle performance, helps you bulk up and gain weight so I pass on this and/or pre-workout which gives extreme energy which I have naturally.

Keep It Off

Play is Medicine
The definition of play is to engage in activity for enjoyment and recreation rather than a serious or practical purpose. When I was a kid, we used to play all the time in so many different ways - slides and swings, climbing trees, riding bikes, tag, hide and seek, swimming, sledding, board games, toys, coloring, etc. We also played sports - softball, baton twirling, roller skating. It's important to play and laugh even as or especially as an adult. Have some fun! Do things for enjoyment and recreation. Maybe it looks the same as when you were a kid - my family has a great time playing Spoons or Apples to Apples especially my Dad. Or maybe it looks different, like going to a concert, show or sports event. Get in some laughter! Laughter strengthens the immune system, boosts mood, diminishes pain, and protects you from the damaging effects of stress.

Self-Reflection Helps Us Heal
I analyze all of my behavior all the time. I try not to be obsessive about it, and I do think it helps me stay on track. Case and point, I gave up Rainbow Nerds for

quite a while. Recently, I started eating Nerd Gummy Clusters and they are even worse for me than Rainbow Nerds! So I asked myself, Why do I have a need to keep going back to sugary candy? The question led me to limit the clusters to a few a day. By counting them, the habit doesn't get out of hand.

I also analyze my loose skin. I tried this skin procedure Neveskin on the front and back of my thighs (my worst looking areas, or at least the top two). It wasn't dramatically expensive, but there were literally no results. I was really disappointed. And I thought to myself, at my age why does it matter? I want to look decent in shorts, but I'm 55 years old. So why do I care? Why does it matter?

Getting measured is another form of analysis I have learned to enjoy. I was curious at Ole Nutrition one morning as they were weighing and measuring another lady so I asked Eva to weigh and measure me and she did. She speaks mostly Spanish, but through the Zumba instructor, told me all of my numbers were good, but my body fat and muscle could be a little better. I need to get the list of the things she measured.

Keep It Off

Anyway, I left and went to another Zumba class in the same strip mall, but it was still on my mind so I went back to Ole after the class. I was talking to Oscar (Eva's husband) about my numbers because he speaks more English. I asked how I could reduce my body fat and increase my muscle. He asked me to explain my daily routine as far as what I eat, drink and exercise so I did. I delicately (well, in my way) explained to him that I start every day with a fiber one bar and 32 ounces of water to keep things going if you know what I mean. What he told me really surprised me! He said I am not eating enough protein…? I swear I exist on mostly protein, but based on what I told him, he said I am not getting enough. I eat a lot of meat, eggs and drink a lot of protein shakes!

We had a very long conversation about Weight Watchers, portion control and my concern that if I increase the amount of food I eat, I would gain weight. He doesn't think I will and that this will help me reduce my body fat and increase my muscle and that they will help me and weigh/measure me weekly or biweekly as I make changes to see what happens. More to come on this.

On my way out, a lady was sitting at a table, having one of the drinks they sell. She stopped me and said she heard my conversation. She said she was a natural healer, and she could sense me and that I need love–self love? She said she wasn't sure I believed in that type of thing or that I may be suspicious since she was a complete stranger, but that she could really sense me while I was there. I don't know how to explain what I experienced other than to acknowledge that she was right about the self love and that I need to figure out what to do about that and that I got teared up a couple of times during the brief conversation with her. On the practical side, she told me that I should buy a body brush and brush my whole body from my armpits to my feet to help with flushing out my system or to keep things going. She explained that she had been in a very bad accident eight years ago and was paralyzed. She had had a similar flushing/going issue and this really helped her. She hugged me and I left, I've thought about it ever since. I'd love to find her and have another conversation.

Keep It Off

Sleep

I have been frustrated many times over the years when things that worked for me stopped working. They used to work, but they don't work anymore. After I get over my frustration and it doesn't take long, I start thinking and reflecting on what is going on in my life at that time. What has changed and what adjustments can I make to keep moving forward. Sometimes your body changes and/or your digestive system changes such as menopause, bowel movements (sorry), side effects of a short or long term medication.

Sometimes the solution is a dietary supplement. Sometimes if you are really honest with yourself you will see that maybe you let your portion sizes creep up a little or your intake calculations (calories, points, whatever) are not as legit as you think. Sometimes you need to really shake up your diet and exercise routines. Sleep and stress are two things you probably didn't think relate to a weight loss and/or fitness journey, but they absolutely do! They can also relate to other health related issues. I will discuss the most common ones. Let's take sleep first. People have different needs when it comes to sleep, but almost all recommendations from all sources recommend 7-8 hours per night for adults.

I think this means good quality sleep. Not the too hot, too cold, can't get comfortable, leg out, leg in, flipping and flopping, mind won't shut down, I have to go to the bathroom, staring at the ceiling, reading for a little while to try to get myself to be tired enough to sleep. My mind just keeps spinning.. 'What is that noise?' This is the kind of sleep that I have suffered with for years. Add that to the fact that I am a high energy person that exercises from 7 to 8 pm most nights and I have a serious struggle on my hands. I gave up many years ago trying to achieve success on my own and started asking friends looking for solutions and did some research. I even talked to my doctor. He recommended Benadryl. Not a great choice for me. Benadryl knocks me out, so that would help me sleep, but it also leaves me feeling super groggy the next day. No thanks.

So at the recommendation of a friend I started taking melatonin as a dietary supplement. It helped some for a while, but not as well as I had hoped. Even so, I still take it every night. It also often gives me really vivid dreams.

At the recommendation of another friend, I tried the Kirkland sleep aid from Costco. She told me she took three or four per night, but I decided to start with just one. The next morning I realized I slept like a rock, but I literally walked to the shower with my eyes closed so it was a little too much for me. So I backed down to half and that works great for me. I like how I take it, get in bed, read for about 30 minutes or less and slowly just drift off to sleep. Now I don't gamble, take my chances or wait to see what happens. I just take my melatonin and half a Kirkland sleep aid and go to bed. I do my best Monday-Friday to be in bed between 9 and 9:30 pm, and I think most nights I get 6 to 7 hours of decent sleep. I still wake up a few times during the night for various reasons.

Saturday and Sunday I don't have to get up early for work so I usually take advantage of that by staying up later at night and getting up later in the morning. I do not set an alarm on Saturday or Sunday. Monday–Friday I get up between 4:30 and 5 am to start work between 5:30 and 6 am. I am a morning person, but thanks to the help of my night time sleeping cocktail and staying up later, I usually don't get up before 8 am on Saturday or Sunday unless I have something specific to do or somewhere specific to be earlier. So on the weekends I think I'm getting at least 8 hours of decent sleep.

I don't know that my night time cocktail is the right thing to do long term, but I don't think it's hurting me in any way and I am getting the sleep and rest that my body so desperately needs. So what happens when you don't get proper sleep? Again all people are different. When I don't get proper sleep, I'm not as sharp and on top of my game as I usually am. Thank goodness my job isn't a matter of life or death. I'm not doing surgery or anything like that. When I don't get proper sleep, I get irritated with things I normally would not and I get irritated much quicker. I may be short with people, less positive, less productive to name a few. I never allow lack of sleep to be an excuse to skip work or my exercise class, but maybe you do? I try not to let lack of sleep impact my choices, to be lazy with my diet or responsibilities, but maybe I'm not as diligent as usual. Stress can impact you, your

Keep It Off

physical and mental health and your relationships in so many ways. Some similar to lack of sleep and some completely different.

Don't Let Go of the Wheel

I know I've already mentioned all the gym closings I've dealt with in the past, but they were a really big deal. Things like this can really throw off your weight maintenance. When Curves closed about seven years ago, I started going to classes at Jordan Valley Athletic Club such as power pump and total body conditioning with Sam as the instructor. I learned from others in the class that Sam was a former champion bodybuilder. I went to Sam's classes every week until Jordan Valley Athletic Club closed about five years ago. A couple weeks ago, my friend and I ran into Sam, owner of Luxe Body Worx which sells luxury handcrafted soaps and products that benefit your skin, health and well being and she was at the craft fair selling her products. We all talked and reminisced for quite a while about our time together at Jordan Valley Athletic Club. We thanked Sam for being a great instructor and for all the things she taught us that stuck.

Keep It Off

Sam was great about making sure each person in her class had the right form when doing different exercises with weights, squats, lunges, planks, etc. Her goal was to make sure you didn't hurt yourself and that you worked the muscles you were supposed to be working and in the right way. When I started going to Sam's classes, I had never really lifted weights before or used some of the equipment we used such as resistance bands, medicine balls, stability balls, etc. So I really appreciate to this day everything I learned in her classes.

When I started, I was using five pound weights and Sam was good at challenging each person and noticing when they were ready and needed a little push to move up to heavier weights. Some of us (me) had to be guided the first time to move up to heavier weights (I would probably still be using the 5 pound weights), but after that knew when we could handle more. I got up to fifteen pound weights over time, and felt comfortable and proud that I was getting stronger.

Sometimes in Sam's class I felt like I was going to die, but that just told me I was working parts I had maybe never worked before and/or they needed more attention. I still had things to learn and everything I was doing was making me stronger. I can still hear Sam in my mind when I am exercising saying your knees should never go past your feet when you are squatting or lunging and your butt shouldn't be in the air when you are planking. I can't explain it in words exactly, but the form you should have when you are doing deadlifts or upright rows. If you ever have an amazing instructor like Sam, listen to everything they say, learn as much as you can, and let them push and challenge you to be your best.

  I meet with my wonderful editor/publisher once a month and we discuss what I wrote last month and bounce around ideas and topics for the next month. Inevitably each month, I will go off and write about whatever inspires me or strikes me when I'm thinking while I'm showering, drying my hair, out walking, working or at other times and often not about topics we discussed. This has been the case for almost a year now. My point here is that I feel very passionate about the topics I write about and I am absolutely thrilled with the concept of sharing my story and possibly being able to help others. I want to give real life information and topics that will be relatable to others. Information worth reading, tips that can be tried out, tested and implemented. Thought provoking information that leads to action.

When I got halfway through the initial writing for this book, I had a month where I didn't feel as inspired and motivated as usual. I was disappointed and worried. I was thinking to myself you were so excited and really wanted to do this! What happened? So, when I next met with my wonderful book lady (that's what I call her LOL), she said well you are about halfway and that happens. It's normal. I was so relieved! I mean I had no idea it was normal. I've never written a book before. We got to talking about the middle and she asked if there could be a middle issue with weight loss. Could it be more difficult to continue when you get halfway? I had to spend some time thinking about that. I'm one of those people that suck at job interviews and immediate responses to stuff. I need time to think and have great stuff hours or days later.

So, here's what I came up with: I'm not sure I knew when I was in the middle because when I started

I didn't have an exact number of pounds to lose in mind. I just know I was severely overweight and facing life long health issues and had to get started. That said, about 40 pounds into my journey (looking back now) was technically my original halfway when I ended up hitting my Weight Watchers goal of 125 pounds and I did have a very difficult time as I felt stuck or plateaued.

This isn't the same as dealing with something as difficult as grief or a divorce, but you will go through similar stages (denial, anger, bargaining, depression and acceptance). It's a process I went through at the 40 pound mark and the 80 pound mark. At least those were the most memorable times. There were many days and times over the years I wanted to scream and throw the scale out the window.

There were many days when I felt sorry for myself and talked to myself: 'Why won't the scale budge? I'm eating better and exercising but I'm no longer seeing results.' I wouldn't let this go on for too long before I was ready to really look at what I was doing (and track/review everything I was eating, drinking and how I was moving my body). 'What changes can I make or adjustments, tweaks, substitutions, modifications will help me move forward or keep going?' 'I guess this is it? The acceptance phase.' Still, I made changes. This was when regular margarine became spray butter and oil became cooking spray. Costco bagels or muffins became eggs and skinny bagels. This was when exercise changed from three nights a week for thirty minutes at Curves only to adding other exercise in.

It bothers me when people say they don't have time. Everyone has time for what they decide is important in life and that's what they prioritize. I know it's hard to juggle everything you have or want to do in your life. You have to decide what is important to you and make sure you prioritize those things and make time for them. And it's okay to put yourself first once in a while without guilt. Your physical and emotional health is important. You can be better for others if you are the best version of yourself. I know this isn't easy and it took me a long time to get here.

Twenty years ago when I started on my weight loss and fitness journey I was working full time as a salaried employee, with a baby boy, considered obese and pre-diabetic. I started going to Weight Watchers once a month, tracking what I was eating, trying to change what I was cooking and eating. Eventually for exercise, going to Curves after work three nights a week for thirty minutes. Yes, I was a new mom and yes, I felt guilty but I was trying to become a better version of myself so I could be a better wife, mom, employee, sister, daughter, friend, etc. After all these years of consistency, I can honestly say that I feel better physically and mentally when I get in some form of exercise - walking in the park or on the treadmill, hiking, going to the gym or a Zumba class. Even if I am alone during some of these activities, I still feel like it gives me more energy when I make time for exercise. I enjoy it in a group or alone. It's worth the investment and guess what? I still have time for all of my responsibilities at home and work as well as time to do fun stuff with family and friends.

    I previously talked a lot about why and how I got fat in the first place. Some of it was how I was raised to eat prior to my parents' divorce. Some of it was living with my mom who worked multiple jobs, didn't eat much at all and didn't really think about food. As soon as I got a job and could buy food and eat whenever I wanted and as much as I wanted I did. Some of it was because I got a car and stopped walking or riding my bike places or going to gym class at school. Maybe some of these things contributed to my weight gain and maybe they didn't? I've never talked to a therapist about this stuff or anything else. Maybe I should? Until my parents got divorced when I was twelve, I had a really good childhood, but from then until I graduated high school at seventeen many things happened that were really not good that could have also contributed to my weight gain. I don't know if I want to share some of those things or not? Some of them only my sister or mom know. Some of them I've never shared with anyone.

    I guess the point here is, there could be or are lots of reasons people get fat. Some of the reasons are psychological such as dealing with stress and different types of abuse. When I was fat, I felt unseen (not even sure that is a word). I don't think like this, but I can understand why some people struggle to lose weight or make an unconscious choice to stay fat as a defense mechanism. They may be thinking, if I'm fat maybe I can avoid attention, protect myself from future abuse, be unseen or unattractive.

Let me just say that I know a lot of beautiful women that are overweight and they may be that way because they love to eat and they are very happy and that is totally fine! Weight management and fitness isn't for everyone. Just like all the advertisements via different formats, there are also so many things that suggest how you should look, but for the most part they are completely unrealistic. Think about all the sitcoms, commercials, magazines, etc. where all the women look like a size 2 with perfect bodies, tans, hair, teeth, skin, nails, makeup and clothes. How many people in your life look like that? How many people in your entire life have you seen that look like that? I'm thinking not very many.

Don't get me wrong, I know some beautiful ladies, but I can't think of many that have all that perfection going on at the same time. It's not realistic. Also, models and actresses have people. LOL. People that do their hair and make up, personal trainers if they are really good, somebody that does the cooking, cleaning, laundry. How many people in your life do

Keep It Off

you know that have any of that? Not very many right? I see all of those things and I think to myself I want to look just like that, but it's not realistic. Don't compare yourself to models, actresses or anyone. I know that's easier said than done because we all do it! Instead of comparing yourself to someone and wishing for some attributes they have, try to become the best version of yourself. Love the skin you're in! Also easier said than done. Some techniques that help me feel better about myself include complimenting others sincerely and often. Accept all compliments given to me as sincere with a thank you and a smile. The other day I was picking up takeout in workout clothes and no makeup. The lady working there said my skin looks amazing? I'm 55 years old and without makeup? My response was thank you very much!

Several years into my weight loss journey, I was still learning (and kind of in denial) about certain foods and what it would take to achieve true success. Maybe I should have known better or had more common sense. For instance, I discovered these Otis Spunkmeyer double chocolate muffins and I whipped out my Weight Watchers calculator to figure out the points. The answer was six! I couldn't believe it. I was really excited. So I started eating these muffins for breakfast and boy were they yummy! Then my weight loss stalled and I was trying to figure out why. What was different? I realize that eating these muffins coincided with my stalled weight loss. So I recalculated the points and I still came up with six using the nutrition label. Then I start analyzing the label. The serving size was half a muffin! The muffin was twelve points! Lesson learned and now I validate and question things, pay attention to the details. Anything that tastes that good and in that portion size is not six points.

If I had to make a list of things I do not like to do, bra shopping would be one of my top dislikes. I used to wait until my bras had been washed and worn so many times you couldn't tell what color they were and they were about to disintegrate before I would go bra shopping. The only time I've had any boobs to speak of was when I was fat or pregnant. When I lose weight, I always start to lose it in my shoulders and boobs first. Don't get me wrong, I like my small A cup boobs. People say with age they sag. Let me tell you, if

Keep It Off

you don't have much they can't go far! Anyway, about twenty years ago I was fussing with my BFF about needing to go bra shopping, how much I dreaded it and whenever I tried them on I looked like Madonna with the cone bra or little torpedos.

My BFF said it couldn't be that bad, she would go with me and so off we went to Kmart. Why Kmart of all places I don't know? So we pick out a bunch of bras and go into the fitting room. I started trying on bras. Let me stop right here and explain that my BFF has really big boobs and a ton of cleavage. She even had to get those girls knocked down years ago because they were killing her back carrying them around, but I'd swear they grew back. Anyway, as I'm trying on bras she says, 'oh my God they do look like cones!' 'Why do you have so much space between your boobs? It's like a whole valley!' 'We are being loud and obnoxious and laughing so hard.' I literally have less than zero cleavage. There isn't a push up bra in the world that can put my open valley together and produce an ounce of cleavage and I'm okay with that. I just don't want cones! We ended up having a great time and I think I did end up with a couple bras that weren't awful.

My point here is, love what you've got. I love my microscopic A cup boobs. I don't have to worry about them jiggling when I exercise or a shirt being too tight across the boobs. Many years later, I bought some padded bras that are quite flattering. My sister even asked me one time if I had something to tell her and I was like what do you mean? She said where did you get those? I laughed and said girl I just got measured appropriately and that is padding. I didn't buy new ones like another family member when she turned 50.

I like to do a lot of reflecting. It helps me put things in perspective, find improvements I can make and continue to grow. It probably sounds corny, but true. Looking back, I realize I was always doing some type of exercise. At the least, walking and listening to music. I never had an issue being active. My issue was with food. Bad food choices–my favorite foods were really bad for me (you might remember me mentioning cheese fries and Chicken Alfredo). My portions were too large - I would eat until I cleaned my plate, if it tasted good I would keep eating, sometimes I would go back for seconds. I swear my 'I'm full' indicator was broken or never worked. I also lacked control, will power and discipline. All of these tendencies are still there. After more than twenty years, it's still a daily battle. Some days are better than others and it's all worth the fight.

About two months ago, my family started fussing that the scale was being erratic and inaccurate, but it seemed to be working fine for me. I use my monthly Weight Watchers weigh-in to help me calibrate my home scale and it's usually within half a pound and it was two months ago. However this past week it also started being erratic for me although I was still hopeful it had maintained its usual accuracy. When I got to Weight Watchers, I saw the poster in the window that said how would you measure success if the scale didn't exist and my current answer is still the same–I don't know because I use the scale to measure success.

Anyway, I was disappointed to discover that my home scale was no longer accurate. It was low by about two pounds and so it was time to buy a new one.

I ordered it immediately on Amazon and received it the next evening. I use the scale to monitor my progress every day and I want it to be as accurate as possible. My last scale was Weight Watchers and so was the new one I ordered. As I was looking through my new scales instructions for use, I found it interesting that it gave advice about using a scale such as: "Important Information Concerning Management of Weight - Your scale is the best tool for monitoring weight. While not the only measure of weight loss, scales are the most popular method used to gauge weight loss success. A scale measures the sum of your total body weight."

It went on to talk about why our weight fluctuates. It mentioned the following factors:
- Salt and carbohydrate intake affects water retention.
- A large meal adds weight short term and can cause water retention.
- Dehydration from exercise, illness, or low fluid intake can result in weight loss.
- Even muscle building can contribute to short-term fluid retention.

- A woman's cycle can cause temporary weight gains and losses.

Digging Up Motivation

I'm going to tell a story that speaks to my determination when I decide I am going to do something. Within a couple months of moving to Utah and doing some local not too difficult hikes, a friend from work and I took a Friday off to hike Grandeur Peak. This would be my first summit hike as well as the longest and most difficult hike to date. Grandeur Peak is 5.9 miles roundtrip with an elevation gain of 2,365 feet. I was born and lived in Delaware for the first 38 years of my life where the highest elevation is 60 feet. Now I live in West Valley City, Utah where the average elevation is 4,300 feet. It was a cold day so we decided to wait until it got to 50 degrees to start the hike. I was wearing jeans, New Balance sneakers, t-shirt, hoodie, a coat and carrying a backpack.

We started the hike and within the first half mile I was sweating profusely and overheated. I am a very vocal person. I say, "Oh my God, I am so hot." "I can't breathe." "I have to get out of this coat." I put the coat in my backpack and we continued. We didn't get very far and I said, "I have to get out of this hoodie." I put the hoodie in the backpack and we continued. I was down to a t-shirt at that point. I said, "Soon I'm going to be hiking in my bra."

I noted the raised eyebrows from my friend who by the way had barely broken a sweat. We cleared the woods and started switching back. I had to stop a lot to catch my breath, drink some water, wipe my forehead and take some pictures. We were making slow progress. About 2 miles in, I realized I had to pee. I held it as long as I could while we hiked, but all the while I was trying to figure out where I could go. I yelled to my friend, "I gotta go now! Where am I gonna go?" He said, "Squat between those two trees." He turned his back to me and watched to make sure no one was coming down the mountain. I removed my backpack, grabbed a couple napkins and squatted between the two trees while looking down the trail to make sure no one was coming in either direction. I did my business and got myself back together. I asked, "What do I do with these (the napkins)?" He shrugged.

Keep It Off

I put them in a plastic Walmart bag and then in my backpack and we kept going.

We got to about 2 1/2 miles and there was snow on the trail. I was completely exhausted.

My friend said we could turn back if I wanted. I said there was no turning back. We kept going. I fell down. I'd like to say I slipped on the snow, but I fall down a lot without any help from the environment. My friend helped me up and asked if I was okay. I said I thought so. He said again we could turn back if I wanted. I repeated that there was no turning back. I didn't care if I had to crawl—I was making it to the top. We kept going. I was beyond exhausted and not sure how I was able to continue. I was starting to get delirious. I grabbed my friend by both arms, looked him dead in the eyes, and said, "Where is the top of this @#$%! mountain?" He said we were almost there. We turned the corner and we were at the summit.

Oops. Everyone at the summit had heard my tirade. My friend said the moment I grabbed him he thought I had altitude sickness and was going to throw myself over the side. He was thinking what he would tell my family if he came back without me. I made it.

We were at the top. The views were incredible! I took a bunch of pictures. We sat on a huge rock ledge and took a long break. It was cold and I put some clothes back on.

 I ate some fat-free potato chips and drank a Smirnoff Ice in celebration (I never said I was smart). He drank a beer. We took it all in and rested. When we were ready, we hiked back down. Going down was so much easier. When I decided I was doing something, I did it. I was all in, whatever it took. I have since acclimated to the elevation/altitude, become a much more experienced hiker, and improved my condition so I wasn't stripping when hiking. I would never drink alcohol on a hike again. Not a good idea. It was water only now with an ice-cold Diet Pepsi waiting in the car. I had invested in hiking shoes with lots of tread, and I had discovered dry fit! Potato chips, even though they were fat free, had been replaced with pita chips, peanuts, and granola bars. And I knew where to go and what to do with the napkins now!

 I am blessed with natural energy and motivation. I'm not sure how you get motivated if it doesn't come naturally. I'll talk about what motivates me and maybe something will resonate or help you figure out what will motivate you. My motivation is different now than when I started my journey. The things that motivated me at the beginning were trying not to become diabetic and refusing to buy a size 20 pants.

The things that were motivating along the way were seeing the number on the scale go down, being able to buy smaller clothes, feeling better. Things that continue to motivate me: successes and failures, setting and achieving goals, challenges, weight gains and losses, finally seeing myself thin when I look in the mirror, music, how I feel after a workout, doing things outside. Maybe an upcoming event such as a wedding and the desire to wear a certain outfit will motivate you to get started? Maybe setting and achieving a small goal you set will motivate you to set another and another and you will just keep going? Maybe going down a clothing size or fitting into or back into

> It doesn't matter how slow you go as long as you don't stop.

something? Maybe seeing results on your body like muscles you didn't notice before? My body is a mess. I mean I've lost 100 pounds so I'm mostly loose saggy skin and stretch marks, but I'm damn proud of the one and a half abs I see in the mirror and my shoulders look damn good too! Maybe compliments from family, friends or strangers will motivate you?

It's important to build people up. When I see people working really hard at the gym or dieting and I see a difference, I make sure to tell them. What comes around goes around can be a positive thing!

Choices, Choices, Choices
I recently realized that I have subconsciously trained myself to make better eating choices. For instance, I have almost completely stopped choosing foods that I love but know are high in Weight Watchers points. It's not that I was eating them on a daily basis or that I cut them completely, but I have significantly reduced them. Some examples: bagels with cream cheese, muffins, hot dogs, cheeseburgers, macaroni and cheese. I used to eat a bagel with cream cheese or a muffin on Saturday mornings, but somewhere along

Keep It Off

the way I stopped doing that. Now on Saturday mornings, I usually eat a fried or scrambled egg with or without salsa, cheese, ham or chorizo and a skinny bagel with spray butter. I don't really miss the bagels with cream cheese or the muffins and once in a blue moon I will still have one. When the weather is good (60 degrees or higher), I like to cook on the grill.

With my busy work schedule, I try to cook as much as I can on Sunday evenings so we can have leftovers as many nights as possible and I don't have to find or make time to cook a decent meal. Usually I grill hamburgers (my son's favorite), chicken always, sometimes brats, hot dogs, carne asada or some combination. Although I love hot dogs and cheeseburgers, I find myself going for the chicken or carne asada almost automatically every time. Is it to avoid the bread (roll)? Is it because I know chicken is a better choice? I'm really not sure. I did have a hot dog with the roll on Memorial Day on purpose and it was delicious, but after that back to chicken. There are some things I haven't and will probably never cut. I get 21 bonus Weight Watchers points per week to use however I want. I mostly use these on weekends to enjoy a larger portion of something, something less healthy than what I eat on weekdays (not that I'm making super healthy choices any day) or special treats I love like pizza or ice cream.

Portion control is a very important thing I learned from Weight Watchers. The amount of food I was eating each day before I learned about portion control was way higher than what I should have been eating or what my body needed. I eat much smaller portions now and I am completely satisfied. I'm not starving at all. Obviously when I first started reducing my portion sizes, I felt hungry in between meals and a little deprived at first. In some time, my body adjusted or I would and still do eat a small snack in between if I feel really hungry.

> I may act like I'm okay but deep down inside I'm hungry again.

Full transparency, I do often feel hungry between breakfast and lunch probably because my usual breakfast is a fiber one bar. When this happens, I internally talk to myself. It's only an hour until lunch,

Keep It Off

can I make it? Most days the answer is yes. Once in a while the answer is no and I have to get a little snack. A lot of times when we get takeout, I order the kids meals! Restaurants put age limits on kids meals so you can't always do it when you eat at the restaurant, but when you are getting takeout, they don't know who you are feeding. I personally think anyone should be able to order whatever you want, but I won't go there! I often find the portion size of kids' meals to be the same as the adult meals, but if the portion is smaller which is what I'm looking for, it is always enough food for me. And not to state the obvious, but kids meals usually cost a whole lot less! I like to tease my son and tell him, you can get the adult meals now and I'll get the kids since he was about 10 years old. The reason I do this is because I know myself. I'm not good at boxing up half and eating half at the start of the meal. I'm not good at only eating half of what is put in front of me. I'm guaranteed to eat more than I need, overeat, tell myself one more bite that actually turns into ten or I end up eating all of it every single thing/time.

      I truly believe you need to have balance in your life. You can't put all your time and energy into one thing long term without falling short or neglecting something else. I have a formula that has worked for me for many years. I have always put work, family and responsibilities including bills first followed by chores and entertainment. A typical week for me looks like this: Monday through Thursday I usually work 6 am to 4 pm. I'm very thankful to be working from home full time since 2018. I eat a fiber one bar with water for breakfast, carnitas or chicken with pita chips and Diet Pepsi for lunch, maybe a little chocolate for a snack and grilled chicken, carne asada or eggs with pita chips for dinner. I try to walk at least 5 miles every day which can be during conference calls, lunch, a quick break or after work.

    At 7 pm, I go to a Zumba class. I'm up by 5 am at the latest to shower. I shower again after Zumba. I'm in bed by 9 pm and usually read for 30-60 minutes and asleep by 10 pm. I do laundry whenever there is enough for a load, usually multiple days a week. I go to the mailbox and through the mail every day. Tuesday mornings I empty all the trash in the house into the primary trash and recycle in the kitchen in preparation for my son to take everything out to the

Keep It Off

cans in the garage and out to the curb Tuesday night for Wednesday pick up. On either Wednesday or Thursday morning depending on who is getting paid, I pay bills and balance my checkbook. On Wednesday or Thursday after work, I check all supplies and make Walmart, Costco or Sam's Club lists. A lot of Fridays I only work a half day. I spend the afternoons lots of ways: doing laundry, taking an extra Zumba class, running errands, going to Costco, cleaning, reading, taking a walk or a combination of several of these.

Friday night is takeout night for dinner and we rotate who gets to pick what we have. Sometimes on Friday night we will watch a movie or a show. Sometimes we will relax or read. Sometimes we go to bed early. Saturdays are mostly for fun. We usually plan a hike or day trip up to 6 hours away. We get up really early to get breakfast at the gas station, usually a donut or breakfast burrito and I get a 44 ounce Diet Pepsi. We hike, bike, walk, sightsee and take pictures. We usually pack snacks and drinks in the car for lunch and then find a place for dinner wherever we are when we get hungry.

Sometimes we get back really late. At least one Saturday a month we stay home. On those Saturdays, I sleep later than usual (around 8 or 9 am). Sometimes I will go to a Zumba class. I usually make eggs and skinny bagels for a late breakfast/early lunch. Sometimes I go shopping, clean, run errands, read on the patio, pull weeds or whatever else that comes along to do. Sometimes on Saturday night we will watch a movie or show. Sometimes I cook or we get takeout. If we are home, I usually eat a bowl of ice cream or we go to the Mexican bakery and get sweet bread to share.

Sunday is family day. I usually sleep until 8 or 9 am, get up and shower, do some extra weekly grooming activities and make a big family breakfast which is more like brunch or lunch. There is always bacon and scrambled eggs with either French toast, waffles or pancakes. I usually talk to my mom while cooking breakfast, finalize my grocery list and wash all the sheets and towels in the house. After breakfast, I pack up any leftovers and wipe down all the counters and tables in the kitchen, then I go to the grocery store.

If the weather is good, I will go for a walk outside and read a book on the patio. Around 4 pm, I

Keep It Off

start prepping for a big family dinner. I will cook as much as I can for a fresh Sunday dinner and plan for as many days as possible so I don't need to cook during the week and I know what I'm going to be eating during the week so I can stay on my plan. After dinner, I pack up the leftovers and wipe down all of the counters and tables in the kitchen. Sometimes on Sunday night, we will watch a movie or a show. I may have a bowl of ice cream or some Mexican sweet bread. Around 9 pm, I head to bed ready to start a new week on Monday. My son has had chores since he was big enough to roll the trash cans down to the curb. He is responsible for the trash, recycling, unloading the dishwasher, running the vacuum cleaner and keeping his room clean. Insert eyeroll here.

If someone is sick, working a weird shift, out of town or unavailable for whatever reason someone else automatically steps in and completes their chores. It seems to work for us and everything gets done. The guys are also responsible for cutting the grass, edging and shoveling the snow. I do all the shopping, cooking, laundry, finances and planning. Everyone has responsibilities, work, and fun. I hope it's a good balance for my family.

Discipline, Know Thyself

If you know what your strengths are, you can use them to achieve your goals. I'm a self motivated, organized, detail oriented planner with a ton of natural energy. I have used these strengths to help with my personal and professional goals as well as everyday life. I used to spend a lot of time and effort trying to improve my weaknesses (lack of patience is one of them) until I took this class at work called Strength Finders. Best class I've ever taken at work. What Strength Finders teaches you is learning how your strengths can overshadow your weaker areas, being well rounded doesn't necessarily lead to higher performance. You can achieve the highest levels of success only when you stop trying to be a little bit good at everything and instead hone what you are naturally best at. Focus less on being well rounded and more on becoming better at what you are already great at. You take an assessment and then get a report of the 34 themes of talent in order based on your responses and focus on the top 5

dominant ones first. Here are my top 5 with a short summary:
1. Achiever–People who are especially talented in the Achiever theme have a great deal of stamina and work hard. They take great satisfaction from being busy and productive.
2. Communication–People who are especially talented in the Communication theme generally find it easy to put their thoughts into words. They are good conversationalists and presenters.
3. Woo–People who are especially talented in the Woo theme love the challenge of meeting new people and winning them over. They derive satisfaction from breaking the ice and making a connection with another person.
4. Input–People who are especially talented in the Input theme have a craving to know more. Often they like to collect and archive all kinds of information.
5. Discipline–People who are especially talented in the Discipline theme enjoy routine and structure. Their world is best described by the order they create.

And to round out my top ten:
- Consistency
- Empathy
- Maximizer
- Individualization
- Analytical

I believe my strengths of self motivation, achiever, discipline, and consistency coupled with a ton of natural energy are what have made me successful with so many of my goals both personally and professionally as well as continuously re-evaluating goals and creating new goals. I also believe slow and steady wins the race and if at first you don't succeed, try try again. It's these strengths and beliefs that have me up really early every morning, getting on the scale, drinking water, watching what and how much I eat and drink, logging everything, working a long hard day and giving my team my all, getting my walking in, having dinner with my family taking care of my personal responsibilities, going to my Zumba class, reading to unwind and getting up the next day to do it all over again!

Keep It Off

Outside of work I took a VIA Character Strengths Survey and my top five strengths came out as: Kindness, Leadership, Honesty, Perseverance and Curiosity. I think these strengths, specifically perseverance (persistence in doing something despite difficulty or delay in achieving success) and curiosity (a strong desire to know or learn something) are what have helped me and continue to help me on my journey.

Vices and Victories
Everyone has vices or addictions or whatever you want to call them. I believe we have them throughout our lives. I think some people have the same ones their whole lives and some people trade one for another, but we always have at least one. I'm a trader. I think about my past and current vices/addictions, evaluate how good or bad they are and if or what I'm going to do, if anything, about them. Many years ago, I smoked cigarettes socially/casually about a pack per week. I decided for me it was a very bad vice and I quit cold turkey. Honestly, I still miss smoking cigarettes sometimes even after quitting more than 30 years ago,

but no plans to ever go back. I'm not sure if overeating is a vice, a lack of awareness, or what, but I have also stopped that for the most part. I still overindulge on occasion. I replaced overeating with Rainbow Nerds (candy) but I stopped overdoing it with the Nerds a month ago. Now my vices are Diet Pepsi and shopping.

I've cut back considerably on the shopping, too. I mean how many pairs of sneakers or leggings and shirts does one woman need? I still buy a lot of books to read and I do eventually read all of them, so maybe this isn't so bad as a vice? I overdo it with Diet Pepsi. I drink more than a 2 liter most days. I know it's not good for me, but is it really so bad? There are definitely worse things in my mind. I don't drink tea or coffee. I don't regularly (couple times and/or drinks per year) drink alcohol. I don't do drugs. So I drink too much Diet Pepsi and buy too many books or shirts? Maybe that's okay? I'll keep thinking about it.

Hobbies

I've had a lot of hobbies throughout my life or interests. Some have come and gone quickly and some have continued to this day. Some I look back and wonder what I was thinking. Some I miss and haven't added back. I started reading books in elementary school and to this day I spend at least 30 minutes per day reading. I primarily read murder mysteries, but I've been known to read true crime, best sellers that are not murder mysteries, diet, exercise and other self help books. I'm always reading something. Sometimes a mystery and a self help book are in progress at the same time. I have loved taking pictures for most of my life. I take pictures of everything: pictures of my son, family, friends, food, flowers, plants, scenery, funny signs or things, etc. I don't think this will ever stop. I have loved to travel and sightsee most of my life also and don't see this stopping until I am no longer able to do it. One of my goals is to visit all 50 states in the United States and I only have 1 left - Alaska. I have been to Canada and Mexico, on a Caribbean cruise to several islands and to the Bahamas. I want to see the Eiffel Tower and after that who knows?

When I moved to Utah 16 years ago, I started hiking regularly and plan to continue as long as I'm able. Here are some things I did for a while, but I either lost interest, was at a different stage/relationship in my life or wasn't good at it: member of the volunteer fire company, bowling on a league, collecting Nascar cards and other memorabilia, rollerblading (I mean seriously? I fall down a lot just walking), counted cross stitch, scrapbooking, making crafts, watching professional baseball, football, basketball. These days I regularly read, walk and go to Zumba as much as I can. I love Zumba and have been doing it for over 12 years. At this point I don't see myself losing interest in it and plan to do it as long as I'm able. What will come next or in future years? Only time will tell.

Pick a Program that Works for You (Diet and Exercise)

Just like my 37 year career at Discover Financial Services, when I first got started at age 18, I didn't know how long I would stay as I wasn't thinking that far ahead. I just knew it was time for a change and it was too good of an opportunity to pass up. My previous job that I started when I was 15 wasn't getting me anywhere after 3 years and 10 cent raises, and I didn't feel valued, respected or taken seriously. I got over $3.00 an hour more to go to Discover. So when I started my weight loss and fitness journey over 20 years ago, I didn't really know how long it would last, if I would be successful or not, but it was time for a change because I just kept gaining weight and I wasn't healthy at all. I don't really like change or constructive feedback, but over the years I've gotten better about both. I still have room for improvement. The difference is I've worked really hard to grow as a person in all things. I no longer hide from or deny my faults or weaknesses. I don't stick my head in the sand. I face it all head on and forge ahead.

    Someone recently told me I'm a pragmatist and nobody has ever told me that before. I always thought and told people I was a realist. So of course I had to Google it and she was right. It's totally me! Pragmatists talk faster than most people, can be very direct and usually get straight to the point. Words that describe people in this category include: action-orientated, decisive, problem solver, direct, assertive, demanding, risk taker, forceful, competitive, independent, determined and results-orientated.

Anyway, if I was going to give advice on starting or how to start a weight loss and/or fitness journey, I would say make a light plan and just get started. Any small step in the right direction is a step even if you have to take baby steps. Don't set yourself up for failure by thinking you can lose a massive amount of weight in a short period of time or you are going to become a 5 day a week gym rat when you are currently sedentary. First acknowledge what you want to do such as: I want to lose weight and get healthier. I want to be more physically active. Then assess what you need to get started.

Weight Watchers worked and still works for me because my diet isn't the healthiest and you can eat whatever you want as long as you stay within your point budget. Also having to go there and get weighed keeps me in line and accountable. Oh and I can't do a diet that limits carbs too much or focuses too heavily on fruits and vegetables. I would quit, fail and/or starve. So assess what kind of eater you are and pick something that will work for you. Do you need an organized program where you pay or a support system like weekly meetings? Maybe a phone app program will work?

There are so many options out there to choose from. What do you need to be accountable to yourself? Maybe a home scale and a weekly weigh-in is all you need. Aim to lose no more than 2 pounds per week. Be kind to yourself as you get started. Set small goals for yourself such as 5 or 10 pounds and no matter how long it takes to get there, celebrate your success. Assess your current activity level and then figure out how you want to start. I started with Curves for women, which is unfortunately no longer in business, because it only required 30 minutes 3 days a week, was low impact and was women only. Maybe you want to walk 15 minutes a day outside or on a treadmill a couple days a week and slowly add a little time as you go. Maybe you want to do some type of streaming videos at home or try some different classes at a local fitness center. Maybe you need a workout buddy to walk with you or go to the gym with you to keep you motivated or accountable. Just take a small step and you've started! If you crave something don't go hog wild, but eat it. Do not deprive yourself.

I know it's hard to find time for exercise or for yourself especially when you have other responsibilities such as children, husband, family, work, household chores or whatever, but take an honest look at how you are spending your time and I promise you can squeeze something in.

Be realistic with your goals and what you chose to do. I mean if you don't like meat, Atkins is probably not a good choice. If you don't want to give up carbs and fruit, Keto might not be the best choice. For exercise, pick a time and activity that you enjoy. I work with a lady that gets up and goes running at 4 am because she has a five year old son, a job, and a husband that goes to work early. That's when she can fit it in and it works for her. I'm a morning person, up by 5 am during the week and start work at 6 am or earlier, but the thought of any type of exercise in the morning or getting up even earlier than 5 am is a nope. It's just not going to happen. I've tried exercising in the morning multiple times (not 5 am in the morning, more like 9 or 10 am) and my body just doesn't respond like it does later in the evening. Experiment or research what may work best for you with a weight loss and/or fitness program. Maybe start with a Fitbit or other app and small daily step goals to get you started.

Make yourself a priority in any small way even if you feel guilty at first. Self care is very important. Just like they tell you on an airplane, to put your oxygen mask on first before helping others because if you run out of oxygen yourself, you can't help anyone else with their oxygen mask. The same goes for self care. You have to help yourself first and you will be in much better shape mentally and physically to help others such as family and friends.

Figure out how you want to calculate your progress. Maybe you weigh yourself before you get started and then weigh yourself once a week thereafter at the same time of day and same circumstances (with or without clothes, same outfit, etc.). Maybe you want to measure specific body parts before you start and measure them again after one month. Maybe you want to measure how your clothes feel (hopefully looser). I have a very sweet thin friend from India who doesn't exercise or need to lose weight and has worn the same size clothes the whole time I've known him, which is about 15 years. His method is if his pants start to feel tight, it's time to cut back. Anyway, once you think you have figured out what you want to try for your weight loss and/or fitness journey, just get started.

Every small thing and baby step counts! Celebrate every single thing! Walked a mile today? Success! Lost one pound this week? Success! Slow and steady wins the race! Make adjustments as you go. Read things–books, articles, magazines and take anything from what you read that you think will help and benefit you and discard the rest. Try different things such as recipes, exercise and again keep what you like and discard the rest. I mean hasn't everyone found what they thought was an amazing recipe on Pinterest, made it and were like nope! I could tell you all about these super cute Christmas cookies that were a huge pain to make and came out looking like snakes or this chicken that had ingredients you didn't think could be anything other than delicious that came out flavorless.

You fall off the wagon badly for one meal, just start again at the next meal. Not seeing the results you want when you expect? Just keep going! Want to throw the scale across the room? Just keep going! You can do it! You can do whatever you put your mind to! Like Dory says in *Finding Nemo*, just keep swimming. Even if you are barely treading water. Find something that motivates you and gets you pumped up. To pump myself up, I can hear this song in my head or listen to it in my car or on my phone. The song is La Copa de la Vida by Ricky Martin and the lyrics that never fail to keep me motivated and pump me up are: Nothing can hold you back if you really want it! Do you really want it? Find your theme song, your quote, meme or whatever will motivate you to keep going! Create a playlist for your exercise. Find what inspires you! Just keep putting one foot in front of the other literally and figuratively.

When You Change, Not Everyone Will Celebrate with You. Celebrate Anyway.
When you go on any self-transformation journey, you have to be doing it for yourself. Not for anyone else. And when people in your life have insecurities, they will make the changes about them because of what they see, think and feel. There will be jealousy.

It's hard to deal with these things when all you are trying to do is better yourself and all you want is for the people in your life to celebrate your success with you and support what you are trying to accomplish. I was literally asked if I was losing weight so I could find a new man. That thought had never entered my mind. I was outright accused of having an affair which was completely untrue. Not the kind of support and encouragement I was looking for. All of a sudden for the first time in my entire life I was weighing less and wearing smaller clothes than some family members. I actually got this comment at one point: "You bitch! You weigh less than I do." It was said in a laughing joking way but…..

> **Let your smile change the world, but don't let the world change your smile.**

Others at the gym didn't say anything, but they would throw me looks now and again. Maybe I was reading into things that were not there, but in my mind I heard them thinking, "Show off," "bet she has never been overweight a day in her life," "skinny bitch." But

Keep It Off

that's okay–whenever we succeed at something, someone somewhere is going to compare themselves to you or question your motives or both. I don't let it bother me. I just look at it like, that's their insecurities, not mine. I can't let it stop me from doing what I want to do for me.

Protein Shakes & Rainbow Nerds

Tricks to Maintaining Your Weight Loss: I Learned the Hard Way So You Don't Have To

Figure Out: What is Your Definition of Overeating?

After more than 20 years and almost 100 pounds, why do I still occasionally find myself overeating? I was doing it again today while working. I wasn't bored, hungry or eating emotionally. Over a month ago, I quit eating Rainbow Nerds candy cold turkey. I had been eating at least one entire box every day which is obviously unhealthy for so many reasons. I want to say it's because when I'm working and thinking I like to be crunching on something as when I catch myself overeating it's usually when I'm working and always something crunchy. It's usually pita chips and most recently pork rinds. Maybe I should try crunching on ice? I need to stop doing this. It's prohibiting me from achieving my ultimate 100 pound goal. Even though I don't feel hungry, maybe I'm not eating enough? I'm

Keep It Off

going to take my own advice - let it go, forgive myself, tomorrow is a new day and my plan is to start over again tomorrow and try to do better.

Weight Loss isn't Just About Weight
Figure out what inspires you not just on a weight loss and fitness journey, but for all aspects of your life - home, family, friends, career, etc. I love to read so I get inspired by books (fiction and nonfiction), quotes, memes to name a few. I read this one book *4 Blood Types, 4 Diets, Eat Right For 4 Your Type* by Dr. Peter J. D'Adamo. Here I was trying to eat wheat bread and brown rice and according to this book, my blood type doesn't handle those things well! I was trying to avoid beef/red meat and according to this book, my body handles red meat very well! Rachel Hollis has four books that really inspire me .She tells stories about her life from all aspects that I can relate to and gives tips and suggestions for each topic/chapter that helped her. She's funny, direct and real. I took many things from her books and I reread them and/or just look at all the things I tagged in the books to revisit. Two things I implemented and still regularly review are writing

down all the things you are grateful for and putting your goals in writing. For the entire month of January 2019, I wrote down three things I'm grateful for. If doing that doesn't inspire and make you appreciate everything and look at things more positively nothing will!

Write Down Your Goals

Also in January 2019, I wrote down a list of seven goals I would like to accomplish as follows:

1. Visit all 50 states - 49 down, 1 to go - Alaska! (Completed in May 2025!)
2. Get down to 115 pounds - I have surpassed this one and set a new goal of 105 so I can say I've lost 100 pounds. This one is a challenge for me, but I keep working on it every single day! I fluctuate between 106-112, but I'm not giving up. I'm so close!
3. Learn to speak Spanish - I'm working on it! I practice at my Zumba classes at least four nights a week. I google translate words and phrases so I can add to my vocabulary. I have a guy on my team at work now whose first

Keep It Off

language is Spanish and I practice with him. I look up song lyrics and translate them into English so I can understand and learn. I practice at Mexican restaurants and markets. Still learning, but in progress.
4. Earn $100,000.00 per year - one of the things you are not supposed to disclose or discuss so I will leave you wondering.
5. Retire from Discover - If I make it to August 29, 2025, I will celebrate 37 years of service at Discover. I have the years of service needed, but not the age and I'm not ready to retire yet. My goal is to make it to the minimum age required to qualify for retirement (February 5, 2025/55 years old) at Discover so I am eligible and any time after that I can retire when I'm ready or when asked.
6. Stay physically active - I want to do this as long as I'm physically able and healthy enough to do so. I have a daily goal to walk a minimum of 5 miles and I'm at 383 consecutive days of achieving this goal as of yesterday. This is my longest streak and I have started over several

times. I go to an hour of Zumba a minimum of 4 times a week and it is my favorite form of physical activity. I also enjoy hiking and I fit it in whenever I can.
7. Visit the Eiffel Tower - Can't wait to do this, but not planning yet. I want to complete Goal #1 first.

I created my goals list in 2019 and have now updated it twice: 2023 and 2025. I've added some new ones and I truly believe writing them down has helped me realize them!

Drink Water

The biggest and best piece of advice I can give you is drink water! As much water as you can handle. Figure out a way to get it down! I've always heard you should drink eight 8 ounce glasses of water per day or half of your body weight in water. So if you weigh 150 pounds you should drink at least 75 ounces of water per day. If you exercise, you will need to increase the amount of water you drink to compensate for what you

Keep It Off

are losing. It's always best to drink straight plain water if you can.

I like my water very cold and I start everyday with 32 ounces of water with ice in one of my two favorite bottles. The first bottle is a hot pink 32 ounce see through Contigo brand. For some reason water goes down quick and smooth when I use this. The second bottle I got as a gift for my birthday. It's Polar Camel brand, pink with my full name on it (including my full middle name), stainless steel, not see through and definitely more than 32 ounces. As with my Contigo bottle, the water goes down quickly and smoothly when I use this and it stays very cold for a very long time. Doing this gets me halfway to my water goal by 7 am.

So in case you missed it my favorite color is pink. And I guess what I'm recommending here is to figure out how to get your daily water intake in however works for you. Maybe a favorite water bottle? Maybe you like your water warm, cold, with ice, without ice, room temperature, straight out of a plastic bottle. Just whatever works for you. I have seen ladies at Zumba with massive size water bottles that are see through and contain their entire days worth of water so they can fill it up in the morning and work on drinking it all day with a goal of finishing by day's end.

Maybe this is what will work for you? This water thing has not always been easy for me. I had to do a lot of tweaking along the way to get where I am now. First I had to stop drinking Pepsi for breakfast, then Diet Pepsi, then stop putting a Crystal Light flavor packet in, then stop using disposable pop top plastic water bottles, then find a favorite reusable water bottle and then add ice. Take however many steps and however long you need to get here. Again, I highly recommend straight plain water but the good news is other drinks count - juice, tea, coffee, soda are all composed mostly of water so drink up. My water with the Crystal Light flavored packet counts!

There are so many benefits to drinking water such as:

1. Prevents Constipation. Enough said.
2. Aids digestion - drinking water before, during and after a meal helps your digestive system to break down the food you eat more easily,
3. Supports kidneys health

Keep It Off

4. Boosts skin health - drinking water plumps up your skin cells minimizing the appearance of wrinkles and fine lines which keeps you looking younger. I've actually received a few compliments on my facial skin and how good and clear my face looks since I've started drinking more water.

5. Makes you work out better - water is good before, during and after workouts. Drinking adequate water before workouts makes you workout longer and avoid muscle cramps.

6. Improves mood - it has been proven that negative mood, fatigue and anger increase when you are dehydrated.

7. Keeps you energized - you need to drink water for your body organs to work properly. It also helps maintain healthy blood pressure and heart rate.

8. Helps you lose weight - drinking cold water helps to raise metabolism which makes your body burn more calories. Drinking water helps your body maintain healthy body weight.

9. Boosts the immune system - water plays a vital role in boosting the immune system.

10. Flushes out toxins - water plays a critical role in keeping your body healthy and skin attractive. Water helps your body get rid of harmful toxins through sweat and urine.

11. Boosts your brain power - drinking water regularly helps you focus, think, concentrate, and stay alert.

12. Prevents headaches - dehydration causes headaches

13. Prevents cramps and sprains - water acts as a natural lubricant for your joints and muscles making them less prone to sprains and injuries.

14. Regulates body temperature - water is essential in regulating your body temperature, your body uses sweat to cool down and drinking water replenishes the lost fluid through sweat.

15. Prevents bad breath - drinking water frequently and after eating significantly aids in washing away oral bacteria and removes food particles that cause bad breath.

16. Good for your heart - drinking water helps maintain proper viscosity of blood and plasma as well as the distribution of fibrinogen thereby ensuring good heart health.
17. Ensures efficient transportation of minerals and nutrients throughout the body - minerals and nutrients dissolve in water making it possible for them to reach all your body parts.
18. It aids in forming saliva and mucus that keeps your eyes, nose and mouth moist
19. Helps fight illness - if you drink enough water daily, you are less likely to suffer from constipation, migraines, urinary tract infection, kidney stones, exercise-induced asthma, hypertension and diabetes.
20. Improves oxygen circulation - water is an essential component of your blood and helps to transport oxygen to every part of the body. It ensures one is happy, energized and in good health as oxygen aids in oxidation and metabolism.

Plan... & Then Stick to the Plan

Plan Your Meals: Anything Can Be a Meal Plan

Meal Planning–many people swear by meal planning and meal preparation. I am one of them! Meal planning and prep can look different for everyone, but it for sure helps you stay on whatever program you are on. For some it's a daily process of deciding in advance what you are going to eat that day and documenting it in some fashion so it's kind of set in stone. For some it's actually buying, preparing and cooking meals in advance for multiple days or a week. Whatever works for you is fine. I'll explain the benefits from my perspective a little later.

Note: my food choices/diet are not the best and I am not encouraging anyone to eat what or how I eat. That being said, my theory and concept are good. So let's talk about meal planning and prep–Kristie style. I go grocery shopping every Sunday with a list. I put all the items I and my family need for the week on the list.

Keep It Off

Either my friend or I get fresh carnitas locally (usually on Sunday once a month or so) and I freeze a couple days worth in individual Ziplock bags. I cook a big family breakfast every Sunday and always make extra scrambled eggs. I also cook as much dinner foods as possible on Sundays in hopes that I can stretch it to Thursday. I usually cook a lot of grilled chicken for everyone, but nobody in my house is on the same program/diet as I am, so they have what they like available to them.

 Caution: I am a creature of habit and could seriously and often do eat the same things every day. It's okay if you want and need much more variety. I always have the following items on hand: eggs, skinny bagels, Fiber One bars, Stacy's pita chips, a bag of salad, a bag of pre-cooked grilled chicken, Diet Pepsi, individual Dove chocolates, fresh carnitas, fresh cooked grilled chicken, scrambled eggs.

 Monday through Friday looks like this: water and a Fiber One bar for breakfast, carnitas, Stacy's pita chips and Diet Pepsi for lunch, grilled chicken, Stacy's chips and Diet Pepsi for dinner. If I need something sweet or chocolate, one or two individual pieces of

Dove milk chocolate. I've started snacking on pork rinds if I need a snack. If I don't have carnitas on hand, I will have leftover scrambled eggs with a skinny bagel, a salad or grilled chicken with some kind of sauce for lunch. If I don't have fresh grilled chicken available, I will make a fried egg with a skinny bagel, a salad or frozen grilled chicken with some kind of sauce for dinner. I also always have pre-made low fat protein shakes on hand. Benefits: I already know what I'm going to eat, it's ready and I have a backup plan. Having a plan and backup keeps me from the other options such as hot pockets or ordering takeout especially if I'm especially busy. It saves time during the week, which is great with my demanding job. It keeps me on my program/diet.

> Chocolate is vital for our survival. Dinosaurs didn't have chocolate and look what happened to them.

I'm not sure which is more difficult, being in weight loss or maintenance mode. I was in weight loss mode for 8 years before I became a Lifetime Member of Weight Watchers achieving my Weight Watchers set goal of 125 and having lost 80 pounds. From a Weight Watchers perspective, I've been in maintenance mode since then, but in my mind I was still in weight loss mode or a cross between weight loss and maintenance mode. Although I reached my Weight Watchers goal, my personal goal was 115. It took me an additional 10 years plus COVID to be consistently 115 having lost 90 pounds achieving my personal goal which took 18 years. So, does that mean I've been in maintenance mode for 3 years because until recently I was still losing a little weight and decided to make a push for 105 so I could say I lost 100 pounds which I've seen on the scale three times now, but not consistently.

Here are my top recommendations, tips or suggestions:

1. Keep a food journal.

Years ago, I would not do my food journal while on any vacations including the week between Christmas and New Year's and I gained back 5-10 pounds. I would also be very lax on the weekends.

So several years ago I started taking my food journal with me on all vacations and started being less lax on weekends. I still enjoy food including treats on vacations, business trips, holidays and weekends, but it's no longer the ridiculous out of control free for all it once was. Now I only gain a maximum of 3-5 pounds which is about half of what it used to be and much easier to get back off. Sometimes just seeing my food journal would remind and help me. Finding ways to be active has helped me a lot. Let me say that years ago while on this weight loss and fitness journey, all of the things I was doing to lose weight and be active would go right out the window as soon as I had a vacation, holiday, special event or business trip. I mean it was ridiculous. It would start as soon as I got to the airport! I mean I haven't even left the city/state I live in yet. I diet (insert a better less cringy word here) and exercise (insert another less cringy word here) all year long and most days of the year so enjoying around the holidays and having exceptions to your plan is absolutely okay, but maybe it doesn't have to or need to be a free for all everything out the window deal. Sorry but I went off course there for a page or two.

Keep It Off

2. Finding ways to be active.
Again on vacations, holidays, business trips my exercise routine would go out the window completely. I try my best to meet my minimum daily Fitbit step count every single day (12, 650) no matter where I am or what the event/occasion is. I always pack a pair of sneakers and exercise clothes (one outfit) for all trips - business or pleasure. Now the sneakers and exercise outfit may not make it out of my suitcase, but they definitely remind me to try and be active while I am away from home and I can never use the excuse that I don't have workout clothes or sneakers with me. Most of the time when I'm on vacation or a business trip, I stay active or as I like to say, get my steps in walking in the airport and the hotel. If you are into it, most hotels have an exercise room and/or a pool. Maybe you can find an activity you love while on vacation such as golf, tennis, hiking, walking on the beach, whatever. Just find ways to move your body. I was recently on a cruise and the ship had a gym and an outdoor jogging track. I'm proud to say that I did use the treadmill in the gym and the outdoor jogging track

for walking and a little jogging multiple times during the week. Progress!

3. Try to keep any or as many possible good habits as you can, or as many good meals as you can.
When I know I have a special occasion, holiday or vacation coming up, I try to be as disciplined as possible a week or two before and plan for the same after so I feel more comfortable enjoying myself fully during whatever occasion it is. Sometimes I try to be good for one or two meals a day while on a business trip, vacation or Christmas break. Most often I'm only successful with one meal a day-breakfast. Sometimes the best I can do by choice of course is to get in my daily water goal, step count or some type of physical activity, but whatever habits or routines you can happily continue during these special occasions will help you get completely back on track after.

I have learned from personal experience that it is very difficult to get back where I was with things after spending a week overeating, having a really delicious calorie experience and a fat-infested dessert every night. Each time it was like starting all over

Keep It Off

again from over 20 years ago, and it would take at least a week of misery to get back into all my regular routines, plus several more weeks of serious hard work to get the weight back off. I decided it was not worth the pain and misery. Now I make a few modifications to the free-for-all I was previously doing during holidays, vacations and business trips, and honestly I'm still enjoying myself. I still feel happy and satisfied and for sure the recovery is so much easier and more pleasant. So to summarize, figure out what good habits and routines you can still do, find ways to be active, and keep a food journal, but still enjoy yourself and allow yourself to celebrate special occasions.

While writing the previous pages, I thought of a story about a dinner at a friend's house several years ago. It made me smile so I knew I needed to share it here. It made me think of so many things such as different perspectives, portion control, how people do and believe so many things in life based on who their parents, family and friends are, how they are raised, where they live, what they are exposed to, etc. I was raised in a food loving family where all events were celebrated with an overabundance of food and usually ended with a big bowl of ice cream. I probably should have said I was raised in an ice cream loving family with people that also enjoyed other food!

Anyway, a coworker/friend invited me to his house for dinner one night. I don't remember what we had for dinner or if after dinner we watched a movie or a Utah Jazz basketball game, but I sure do remember dessert. We were having ice cream for dessert. My friend gets out cereal bowls but a lot bigger than the ones I have, and proceeds to put one ball / scoop of ice cream in each bowl. I was thinking what the hell? I guess I should mention that I am a very direct, outspoken, not shy at all person.

Don't get me wrong. I would never be purposely rude or hurtful with my communication and I do sincerely care and think of other people's feelings always. In my mind, I may be thinking mostly what the hell or worse, but most of the time those are not the words that would come out of my mouth. So I said, that's it? And my friend said, what do you mean? And I looked down into this huge bowl with one scoop of ice cream rolling around in it and I said one ball of ice

Keep It Off

cream that's it? and I started to laugh hysterically and he laughed too!

When we both stopped laughing, he said you can have more if you want. My family always serves at least four balls of ice cream per person to the kids and more for the adults. To me, one ball of ice cream was like an insult or an enforced diet! LOL. That's probably why he has always been thin and never had a problem with his weight! And guess what, one scoop of ice cream is the correct and recommended serving size!

I know, right? If you had tried to serve anyone in my family one scoop of ice cream for dessert, they might have asked what kind of cake we were having or thought you must have lost your mind! Balls of ice cream didn't roll around in bowls with my family! And you would not see the bottom of the bowl either! The normal serving size of ice cream in my family was more like four balls and once we made sure everybody got their bowl of ice cream, you could have another scoop or another bowl if you wanted it! Ice cream didn't get freezer burn in my family!

My grandfather, dad and two uncles would have heaping bowls of ice cream with way more than four scoops and multiple different flavors too! I bet we had four half gallons even for just a regular family dinner and multiple different flavors. There would always be chocolate and butter pecan for sure! Anyway, apparently my friend's family fully understood/grasped portion control way before that term was a thing while it took me a lot longer to grasp the concept and my family well...

> There is always room for ice cream.

Dedicated or stupid? I think I've written on this topic before. I am very dedicated and committed to my exercise routine and goals and I try to live and breathe by "no excuses". I am not perfect and I'm not talking about dieting or food right now. I'm talking about exercise plans, routines, and goals. If today is Tuesday and on Tuesday nights at 7 pm I take a Zumba class, then I am at Zumba on that day and that time. Period. One night I got an Emergency Alert from the National Weather Service on my phone: Snow Squall warning until 7:00 PM MST some time after 6 pm. I thought,

Keep It Off

'Okay, it's snowing in Utah. Big deal.' So at 6:40 pm as usual I got in my car and was on my way. I did think to myself maybe I should have left a little sooner and I did check Facebook posts for cancellations. I didn't see any. At 6:51 pm I got a text from an instructor that said he didn't think there was going to be a class due to the weather and my response was 'I'm on my way.' A few minutes later there was a post that the class was cancelled, but there was a class across the street so I went there. I arrived at 7:01 pm and was the only one there for Zumba. I asked the lady that worked there if there was going to be class and she didn't seem sure. I said I would wait a few minutes. I'm not sure she understood. There may have been a language barrier between her limited English and my limited Spanish. While I was waiting, I was getting my steps in and searching for somewhere else to go for a class.

After waiting until 7:15 pm and I was the only one there (there wasn't even an instructor), the lady finally said, "No class tonight." For exercise, I usually have a plan A & B that are solid and a tentative plan C. If all of these fail, I will give in and go home. But that night I headed to a class that started at 7 pm at a Vasa gym. I'm a member and can go to any Vasa location. I figured if I got there by 7:30 pm I could get at least 30 minutes of a class in. At 7:25 pm, I got a text from the instructor from the place I left 10 minutes ago that she was there so I went back. We started at 7:40 pm and ended about 8:15 pm so I got at least 35 minutes of a class in and I did not let the weather (snow) or a cancellation stop me or become an excuse to not exercise.

Maybe I'm stupid, but I like to think I'm dedicated. The roads were truly not bad and I was not in any danger or putting my life or the lives of others at risk. Maybe I'm less cautious than others? I must be if I'm the only one that showed up for class at two different places! Each person has to decide for themselves if they are truly not showing up for exercise because they are concerned about driving in the snow or whatever they tell themselves in each different situation or if it's a convenient excuse to get out of exercising that day. I have routines, plans and goals. No excuses!

Part of maintenance is knowing I will have to have some type of exercise plan for the rest of my life although I'm sure it will change over time. Part of maintenance is knowing I will have to have some type of daily monitoring of portion control and intake of food and drinks for the rest of my life. Part of maintenance is knowing I will have to monitor my weight using the scale regularly although maybe not as many times on a daily basis as I do today. I am about 20 pounds under my Weight Watchers goal of 125 and I planned it that way on purpose to allow myself some wiggle room. I mean I'd like to think I'm a spring chicken who can continue to walk at least 5 miles every day and attend 4+ Zumba classes a week at the same intensity, but I am 55 years old. Who knows what I will be capable of in the future? And if I can't burn as many calories exercising as I do now, I would have to reduce my food intake or I will start to gain weight so I built in a little wiggle room.

From my perspective, weight loss and fitness go hand in hand. You can be thin, but not fit or healthy. You can be fit, but overweight and maybe healthy, but probably not. So you work on both and either start both together or start one and when you are ready add in the other. I started with weight loss and when I was ready incorporated physical activity. Now in maintenance it's like a balancing act to keep everything steady as I navigate through each and every day of my life - the scale, what I eat and drink, physical activity, along with family, work, friends, health, stress etc.

Having a weight loss and fitness journey will have a positive impact on your health in so many ways. For instance, when I had scheduled a surgery on my neck to resolve nerve pain in my left arm, one of the first questions I asked the surgeon was how long do I have to stop my Zumba? And when and what exercise can I do post surgery? Even before the surgery, I was already making a modified exercise plan until I could get back to my usual. I mean I could lay around in my pajamas for weeks eating ice cream out of the carton and use surgery as an excuse, but I had worked way too hard for that.

The week I was having surgery on my neck, February 23, 2024, I knew I should be thinking about my recovery and taking it easy, but that's just not me. Even when I was seriously overweight I was very active and couldn't sit still. So the first things I asked the surgeon about were:

- Missing work (I haven't missed work since I was on maternity leave and my son is now 24 years old)
- Having an incision/scar on the front of my neck (I never considered myself a vain person but maybe I am)
- Not being able to eat (one of the side effects is difficulty swallowing and I swear I haven't missed a meal my entire life)
- Not being able to go to Zumba for 4-6 weeks or do much exercise. Zumba is my stress relief, my therapy, my getting out of the house (I work from home), my way of getting out socially, my fun/happiness that I look forward to at least 4 nights every week

Join A Program that Works for You and Stick To It
I've been doing Weight Watchers for about 22 years and I can attest that it truly works. It works if you are trying to lose weight and if you are trying to maintain your current weight. There are so many things I love about Weight Watchers and I have spoken to many of them while writing (and to anyone that will listen).

What I love the most is that you can eat whatever you want as long as you stay within your points budget. If you want a weight loss plan that you can go the distance with long term, Weight Watchers is it. It's scientifically proven that restrictive diets don't work and there are no foods you cannot have with Weight Watchers.

I've thought a lot about other weight loss plans, researched and explored them too so I ask: Can you really give up carbs forever? Can you really have only two meals a day forever? Can you really do those other food restrictive plans (SlimFast/Shakeology - a shake as a meal/meal replacement, or no sugar or fruit or whatever) forever? Can you completely cut or attempt to avoid whatever those plans are telling you long term? If you can, good for you! I can't. Weight Watchers works for me and suits me best because I practically exist primarily on meat and carbs. Atkins would work perfectly for me if it wasn't for the low carb part. Same with Keto. Can you really eat those pre-packaged meals forever like NutriSystem or Jenny Craig?

Keep It Off

You could probably say the same thing about any/all diets, weight loss plans, restricting of food (or whatever wording doesn't make you cringe) that would work perfectly for me if it wasn't for "fill in the blank". You don't have to say that about Weight Watchers! Weight Watchers works for me because my diet is a mess (a work in progress?). I don't eat any fruit and very few vegetables. Except lettuce and potatoes, any vegetable that I do eat has to be blended until it is completely smooth. I believe the settings on my blender are puree and liquefy. People decide to start a weight loss plan or program for many different reasons - want to fit into a wedding dress, want to look good for a specific special event, want to fit into smaller old clothes they kept, want to try to avoid taking medication or a medical diagnosis or just improve their health in general.

Remember Why You're Doing This
In addition to these, there are many scientific based benefits to losing weight.
1. Lowers risk of diabetes - being overweight increases your risk of type 2 diabetes and it is

20 times more likely in people with a BMI over 35.
2. Improved sleep and energy - losing weight improves breathing and sleep apnea. Better sleep at night boosts daytime energy. Physical activity can help you sleep better. Getting more sleep helps support weight loss by decreasing blood sugar, blood pressure and your appetite.
3. Lowers blood pressure - research shows that losing 5 percent of your weight can normalize your blood pressure.
4. A healthier heart - excess fat causes high cholesterol and when combined with high inflammation, creates an environment where artery-clogging plaque can form easily.
5. Reduced risk of cancer - excess body weight contributes to about 12% of all cancers.
6. More interest in sex - did that get your attention? Being overweight can impact blood flow, hormone levels, and other functions which play a key role in your sex drive. Losing weight has been shown to improve your libido and ability to orgasm. Wow alright.

7. Less achy joints - reducing body fat can lower the physical stress on your joints and not just knees. Pain can pop up in joints all over your body.
8. A better mood - rates of depression are twice as high in people with obesity than those considered healthy weight. Research shows that people who lose 5% of their body weight report feeling generally happier and better about themselves overall.

When you lose weight you can reverse the negative impact it has on your body and that doesn't take long to happen. Experts say losing just 5% of your body weight can make a significant difference. I'm no expert, but I'm living proof that this is absolutely true. When I got pregnant, I weighed 205 pounds and ended up with gestational diabetes. Although I had started on my weight loss journey almost immediately after my 3 month maternity leave, it took quite a while for me to start losing weight because I had so much to learn about portion control, food choices, etc. Anyway I was diagnosed as pre-diabetic (fasting blood sugar level

100-125, under 99 is normal, over 126 is diabetic). I worked really hard on my weight loss journey and started my fitness journey. Within a year, my fasting blood sugar level was 99 or less and has remained for over 20+ years. Diabetes avoidance and this was after losing just 5% of my body weight which is what Weight Watchers encourages as one of the first goals you should set for yourself.

Set a Reasonable First Goal

When you first join Weight Watchers one of the first goals they suggest is losing 5% of your body weight. If you set out to lose 5% of your body weight (provided you have that much to lose) here are some tips on how you can achieve this goal:

1. Start tracking - tracking is the cornerstone of the Weight Watchers program for good reason - it works! Tracking what you eat can make you more aware of your food choices, make you less likely to eat mindlessly and make you more accountable.

2. Handpick your support system - the more support you get from friends and family, the more weight you're likely to lose.
3. Prioritize activity - researchers have discovered that being active is the single greatest predictor of who keeps weight off and who doesn't. Small steps can make a big difference - go on a 20 minute walk, use a fitness tracker to log steps (have a goal in mind), sign up for a new fitness class that you've always wanted to try.
4. Manage stress - because it can trigger higher levels of cortisol and a desire to eat comfort food. Chronic stress can make it harder to lose weight.
5. Improve your sleep - when you don't get enough sleep, you have higher levels of the hunger hormone ghrelin and lower levels of leptin, which is linked to feeling full. Feeling tired can also make it tougher to find the motivation to exercise. One of the best things you can do for sleep is to have a set schedule, meaning you go to bed and wake up around the same time every day (weekends included).

Show Up for Your Weight Loss Journey
I remember one night my stomach was feeling off and I had an accident on my way to Zumba class. I don't want to be too graphic or TMI (too much information), but seriously thank God for panty liners! What do you do in these types of situations? Turn around and go home? Nope, not me. I drove on to the Zumba class and went straight to the bathroom to assess the situation. Also thank God no one was in there! It was a one toilet/one person bathroom. I was thinking maybe the situation wasn't as bad as I thought. It was actually worse. I was absolutely mortified. I probably should have gone home. I ended up washing my underwear out in the sink and putting them in the back pocket of my purse. I washed the spots on my leggings out in the sink with soap and water and put them back on. Thank God my leggings were a dark color. I made sure the bathroom was totally cleaned up and I proceeded to take my Zumba class. I learned I like Zumba without underwear!

I'm like Michael Jordan, but at an ordinary level. He was extraordinary. How many times was he sick or hurt, but went back out on the court and kept

Keep It Off

going, kept pushing himself? How often did he fail, but he just worked harder and kept going? I had a Center Manager years ago that had weekly centerwide meetings and he had a lot of good messages. One of them was you can't be great if you aren't here. First you have to show up. He was speaking about attendance at work, but it applies to so many other things in life. You have to show up at the gym or your exercise classes. When I was overweight and inactive, I used to get sick all the time - sinus infections, bronchitis, etc. Since I've lost weight and exercise regularly, I hardly ever get sick.

You have to show up for your weight loss journey. You have to keep showing up. You have to be consistent and dedicated. You have to overcome obstacles. Don't let them get in your way. It's okay to fail not just once, but over and over again. You have to learn from your failures. You have to push yourself, challenge yourself. Michael Jordan has many famous quotes, but this is the one that always sticks with me: 'I've missed more than 9,000 shots in my career. I've lost almost 300 games. Twenty-six times I've been trusted to take the game winning shot and missed. I've failed over and over and over again in my life. And that is why I succeed!" Be like Mike! No excuses! My motto!

Embrace the Boring: Routine is Your Friend
If I ever had to be under surveillance (yes I have seen too many movies and read too many crime novels), boy do I feel sorry for those guys. They would be bored to tears and ready to quit!

Day 1 Sunday - subject sleeps in as during the week she gets up between 4:30-5 am for work, Subject gets up between 8:30-9 am, takes a shower and does some extra weekly grooming activities (use your imagination), separates the laundry, and starts a load, at 10 am subject calls her mother and talks to her while cooking the usual family breakfast. Every week there will be scrambled eggs and bacon (because the subject's son doesn't like any other style of eggs or breakfast meat). There is a rotation of waffles, pancakes and French toast. After breakfast, the subject puts away leftovers and condiments, straightens up the kitchen and finalizes the grocery list. Between 11:30-12 pm, the subject goes to Walmart, gets everything on her list and checks out. The subject puts groceries away. The subject makes sure to complete her daily step goal by walking inside or outside. The subject puts laundry away. Around 2 pm, the subject gets Diet Pepsi and pita chips and sits down to read her latest murder mystery. Around 5 pm, the subject cooks dinner. After dinner, the subject puts away leftovers, washes dishes and cleans the kitchen. The subject reads or watches a movie, gets clothes ready for work, sets alarm and gets in bed around 9 pm, reads for approximately 30 minutes and goes to sleep.

> If I say "I'm hungry," we've got about 27 minutes until I'm a different person.

Day 2 Monday - subject gets up between 4:30-5 am via alarm and takes a shower. After she is done getting ready she goes downstairs, fills up her 32 ounce water bottle, grabs her Fiber One bar, takes her morning pills and goes back upstairs to start work. The subject works until about 10:30 or 11 am and then takes a break for lunch. She always has Diet Pepsi and pita chips usually with some type of protein - carnitas, grilled chicken, an egg. While eating her protein, she checks her work email and instant messages, personal emails, Facebook and Messenger. While eating her pita chips, she reads her current murder mystery. After lunch, the subject continues to work until 4 or 5 pm. The subject makes sure to complete her daily step goal by walking inside or outside. The subject heats up leftovers for dinner and takes her evening pills. Subject takes two Zumba classes on Monday nights - 5:30 and 7 pm. After Zumba classes, the subject showers and takes her bedtime pills, gets clothes ready for work, sets alarm and gets in bed around 9 pm, reads for approximately 30 minutes and goes to sleep.

Okay, I apologize if you were bored reading that last section, but the purpose of the story was to talk about the importance of routines and consistency. Slow and steady wins the race. Routines and consistency get results.

There will be deviations from your routines and that is okay and expected, necessary, etc. Just try to maintain your routines and consistency whenever you can, as many days as you can realistically, as many

Keep It Off

meals as you can realistically, as many events as you can. Make these routines the rule knowing there will be and allowing yourself exceptions and enjoying them guilt free. You can also have a bad day knowing there is another chance to try again tomorrow! Always try to start each new day on the right foot!

Holidays are Going to Derail You, At Least a Little Bit. Be Ready.

Everyone has a time of year that is hard for them from an eating and exercising perspective. Most people would say it's between Thanksgiving and New Year's, and that is a tough one for sure. Somehow I am able to get through it in decent shape. The time of year I struggle with is the first couple weeks of February. Since we live in Utah, we've started celebrating Dia de la Candelaria on February 2nd. There is a lot of history behind the day as well as religious significance, but we use it as an excuse to eat tamales. February 5th is my birthday and we usually celebrate by going out for a meal and some type of dessert is involved.

Next is the Super Bowl. The Super Bowl for me isn't all about the game. It's more about the company, food, National Anthem, commercials and halftime show. For some reason, I always feel like there should be chips and dip for Super Bowl - salsa with tortilla chips, sour cream and onion dip with potato chips or both. When I lived in Delaware, they had this Helluva Good sour cream and onion dip that was awesome. They don't have it in Utah and I sure do miss it. In my mind, there should always be chicken for Super Bowl with different sauces. Bottom line, artery clogging, high calorie bar food.

    Next is Valentine's Day. I buy a lot of candy and make Valentine's bags for my guys, dinner, but we've started getting a heart shaped pizza at home. Sometimes I get candy and I usually end up eating candy. Then finally there is President's Day weekend. Sometimes we go out of town which makes it harder to stay on my weight loss and fitness journey. If we don't go out of town, it's like a regular weekend with an extra day off from work. I guess what I would say is that I do my best to follow my exercise plan consistently, maybe even doing a little extra if I can fit it in. I take one meal at a time and do my best to stay on my plan for as many meals as I can. All of the events I mentioned are things to celebrate with family and friends and I want to enjoy each and every one without a huge weight gain or setback in my progress. I love food and I love to eat. I just need to balance it out.

Don't Forget the Birthday Cake
I know I've mentioned that one of the best things about Weight Watchers is that you don't have to give up any food item or group. You can eat whatever you want as long as you stay within your daily and weekly points budget. And to confirm it's true with actual proof, I got an email from Weight Watchers on my birthday (February 5th) which says: Happy Birthday Kristie! Celebrate your special day with cake, laughter, and friends - and did we mention cake? No birthday is complete without it. If that isn't confirmation and proof I don't know what is?! I bet you aren't supposed to have cake at all on the keto diet, Atkins, etc. I can't think of another weight loss plan or program that allows and encourages you to eat all foods - no restrictions! Weight Watchers does not know I am

writing any of this and I am not being paid for any of this free advertisement. It works!

Forming New Habits Takes Time: Use Reminders
Does anyone besides me find it difficult sometimes to make a new habit stick or remember to do something? About a month ago, I started having to take a pill at noon every day. It's for pain so you would think I would remember, but no. For several days, I completely forgot until it was time to take the next one, I started to hurt or a couple hours later. I had to put a daily reminder in my phone! I'm still using it! Am I ever going to get it without a reminder? Supposedly it takes 21 days to form a habit, but research has shown that is just a myth. In a study published in the European Journal of Social Psychology, researchers found that it takes an average of thirty days for a new behavior to become a habit. So that new exercise routine you just started and/or that new weight loss plan you just started, be patient, give yourself some space and grace.

As I gather topics to write about, I save ideas as reminders in my phone as I think of them so I don't

Keep It Off

forget. A couple weeks ago, I put a reminder in my phone to write about this place I started going to for Zumba on Wednesday nights and random other days. Here are the notes I took: Ole Nutrition - atmosphere, staff, protein shakes. I have been working through my topics and planned to write about it tonight. How convenient that it's Wednesday and I had an even more amazing experience there tonight. Since the first day and every single day that I have gone to Ole Nutrition, the staff which consists of a husband and wife and two young guys, has greeted me using my name and made me feel welcome. They always smile and speak to me in English or Spanish as I think we are practicing on each other. I started going here because I followed one of my favorite instructors, Erika Leon.

    What I learned is the group of ladies plus Chris, Erika and the staff create this fun, respectful high energy atmosphere that makes you keep coming back. I've gone to many Herbalife locations to do Zumba, but this one by far is the best hands down. Plus they make the best chocolate protein shake I've had at any Herbalife location. It's as good as a naughty shake you may get at a fast food burger place and it's healthy!

Tonight was extra special because it was decorated for Valentine's Day, everyone was wearing red, and Erika gave each person a small bag of candy. Eva gave everyone a healthy Herbalife donut. Chris and his mom gave everyone a piece of homemade pie and Erika did a raffle for Zumba shirts and other stuff with enough items so everyone was able to get something. It was really nice.

Time to Get Started

Take Advantage of Peer Pressure

Peer Pressure is a real thing with many things in life including a weight loss and fitness journey. Sometimes it's hard to stand your ground and be strong when faced with a food you love or an activity that impacts your workout schedule and includes food like a double whammy. I'm a very social person but I've had to be less social on occasion to keep with my plan and goals. I've missed a lot of events and activities and sacrificed a lot but for my personal well being. I think it has been and will continue to be worth it. Sometimes family can be the worst at tempting or pressuring you especially if they are not on the same journey as you. I'm usually head down and successful Monday through Friday but not so much on Saturday and Sunday. I'm working on it but I'm much more vulnerable on the weekends and I often cave in eating things I try to avoid and overeating too. On Friday nights, we get takeout and when it's someone else's turn to pick it's usually pizza or hamburgers and French fries.

Perseverance is the Name of the Game
One night before my surgery, I was driving 20 minutes from home for my monthly Weight Watchers weigh-in, and my mind was spinning. Is my scale accurate? Wow it feels so warm already and it's only 8:30 am (78 degrees). Do I feel good enough to go to a Zumba class today? I had found out the pain in my arm was from 2 severely pinched nerves in my neck, and between medications and IBS my stomach was off. Add to that my left arm was throbbing, but I really wanted to go. If I went to Zumba, should I take Rocio or Diana's class? I'm telling myself - you got this! Go! I don't miss work unless I literally can't get out of bed. The last time I missed work was for maternity leave and my son is 24 years old. I feel the same way about my Zumba classes. I don't miss Monday through Thursday unless there is an event I can't avoid or an emergency. I have gone to work and Zumba with pain and not feeling well and I will continue to do so as long as I am able. I didn't always go on Saturday but today I wanted to go. This is my usual self-talk to push myself to do what I promised myself I would do.

Keep It Off

Do Crazy Fun Things Sometimes
Earlier I was talking about how I tell myself I'm a badass at Zumba and I actually do the same thing when I'm hiking and whether it's true or not in the moment or hours however long it takes to complete a class or a hike, I believe it. On hikes it motivates me and keeps me moving forward. Most hikes have a destination or a reward - a view, waterfall, lake or the hike itself is rewarding with scenery, wild flowers, wildlife and it feels good to push your body to reach the destination and return after completing the hike. Some hikes are quite difficult due to the length and/or elevation gain. Nothing keeps me moving, especially uphill like my inner voice saying you are a badass.

  You've got this. Look at all the people you are passing. I don't really know if I am a badass at anything, but in my mind I am and that's all I need especially when I've hiked a mile downhill and I'm looking at the steep mile climb back up the hill. I prefer hikes that are mostly uphill on the way and downhill on the way back so you get the hard work done first. Inevitably I fall down while hiking (see stories about me falling down a lot) and even then as

I'm getting back up and continuing on I tell myself look at you, you are seriously a badass. You fell, hurt yourself, got back up and kept going. I also tell myself when you get back to the car, there's an ice cold Diet Pepsi in the cooler!

I have this friend from Mexico that might just be as ridiculous and unrealistic as I am, but he has helped me achieve some bucket list items and made me a more spontaneous person which is completely out of character for me. He's helped me make some of my goals and dreams a reality and we've done some pretty ridiculous, awesome, fun things together. I'm not sure what this has to do with a weight loss and fitness journey, but maybe I can make a connection somehow.

Here are a few examples. For about 20 years or more, I dreamed of going to the Balloon Fiesta in Albuquerque, New Mexico. I told my friend about it months in advance and how we had gone to some small local ones, but I really wanted to go. So on Friday afternoon before Balloon Fiesta started on Saturday morning we decided we were going. We packed everything up, printed tickets we ordered online and headed out! We drove through the night

Keep It Off

taking turns and arrived at the event about when the gates opened at 4:30 am. We changed our clothes in the car and went to all the morning activities which were amazing and incredible, but ended at about 8:30 am. The evening activities don't start until about 5:30 pm so we had a lot of time to kill. We found a great breakfast place called Weck's, we went to see the Rio Grande, a park, Old Town, etc. We went back to Balloon Fiesta for all the evening activities including the awesome fireworks at the end. And then it was over and we had nowhere to stay! All the hotels during Balloon Fiesta are at least double the regular price and sold out. So we started towards home. Finally after a few hours we found a cheesy motel with a vacancy in a town called Cuba. We got up the next morning, asked for a recommendation for breakfast, ate at this amazing place called Presciliano's and drove home!

My friend from Mexico and I love Daddy Yankee. Many of his songs are part of every Zumba class I've ever been to. He was having a farewell retirement concert across the US, but not making a stop in Salt Lake City. The closest city he was playing in was Las Vegas. The tickets were pretty expensive.

We hemmed and hauled on whether to go or not. We decided on a Friday night we were going to the concert on Saturday. I got the tickets booked. We got up early Saturday morning, drove to Las Vegas (about 6 hours), went to the North Premium outlets (we also love outlet and bargain shopping and I tell everyone I am the Queen of Under Armour), ate at Tacos El Gordo (they have the best al pastor tacos), went to Premium South outlets, changed our clothes and freshened up in the outlet's bathroom and went to the concert. The concert was incredible. Best concert I've ever been to so far! After the concert we drove down the strip and all the way back home. These are just two examples. There are several more and we have a big one coming up at the end of the year.

Manage Your Stress
Stress can impact the amount and quality of your sleep. Recommendations from all sources say to minimize stress. For most, easier said than done. Stress can come from work, family, friends, relationships, situations, health, and many other things. So what can you do to limit stress? My exercise class is a huge

Keep It Off

stress reliever for me (Zumba) and that is one of the reasons I go as many days a week as I can. I do my absolute best not to miss a class Monday-Thursday nights. Try not to worry, or stress about things that are out of your control. This is a tough one for me that I am still working on. I mean I honestly don't understand what people mean when they say don't take things so seriously or don't take things so personally. It's like saying I should stop being me or stop breathing. These are all things I am personally working on so I am not going to be much help here. Sorry. I guess I would say try to be as healthy as you can in every way you can, take care of yourself, do things for you, make yourself a priority. Another stress reliever for me is being out in nature, hiking, taking pictures and sightseeing. It's especially good in places where there is no cell service so you can completely unplug with no disruptions or distractions fully enjoying the scenery all around you. Find something that is a stress reliever for you and do it as often as you can. And I don't mean eating! I mean

> Balance what you eat, drink and do.

eating can be an enjoyable stress reliever, but it is not going to help you with a weight loss journey (quite the opposite and can actually lead to more stress for obvious reasons). And stress eating is usually not pigging out on broccoli or baby carrots! More like chips or the whole pint of ice cream like you see in the movies.

Mentally Rehearse to Prepare for Exercise and Eating Right (Even on an Ordinary Day)
Another very important tip for success is to be prepared. Back before I started working from home about seven years ago and for all the years I went to Curves, I packed a bag for my workout and took it to the office with me. The goal was to go to Curves Monday, Wednesday, and Friday or at least 3 days a week. I would go immediately after work so there were no excuses. Do not go home, do not start a load of laundry, sit down in front of the TV or tell yourself you don't feel like going to the gym tonight. Now that I work from home and my workouts have changed to later in the evening, I wear my workout clothes as my outfit for the day. There are a few exceptions: if I have

Keep It Off

to be on a video call, I go to the office or I'm meeting for a business lunch which are rare. So after showering and getting dressed in the morning, I'm already ready for Zumba and in the right mindset. I'm also ready for a quick walk at lunchtime or in between meetings if my schedule allows. Lunch for me is usually pre-cooked grilled chicken, eggs or carnitas Monday through Friday. Dinner for me is usually pre-cooked grilled chicken or eggs at least Monday through Thursday. Another way I make sure I'm prepared is by taking a water bottle, other cup, or small cooler with me containing bottles of water and/or diet sodas in it and a decent snack with me wherever I go. I might just be going shopping for a couple hours or I could be on an all day trip, but I try to always be prepared. Unprepared, I will end up at a gas station or a fast food place making bad choices (picture a donut or muffin, burger and fries or who knows what) which I will probably regret later. So try to be prepared for workouts and food and avoid excuses to miss your workout or make bad food or drink choices.

Expect to Be Frustrated Sometimes
Do I get frustrated, irritated, want to throw the scale across the room, quit and eat a huge chocolate chip cookie? Absolutely! Do I quit or eat the cookie at that moment? No, absolutely not. I let myself have my moment (usually just a few minutes, sometimes longer) and then I get over it and move on. I rededicate myself to the cause and try to figure out how to make today and the next measurement on the scale better. Remember I get on the scale every day several times a day. It's a journey and a lifestyle change. It is one day at a time with the opportunity for a restart every single day. There will be days to celebrate, days to reflect, days to be frustrated. There will be days where you plan to eat a huge chocolate cookie or whatever special treat you look forward to, but don't let it be on the day you are very frustrated and want to scream, quit and eat.

On those days, you need to stay true to your strength, will power and dedication to your plan. Do not give in on those days. Let yourself have your moment whatever that looks like for you and then keep going. Sometimes on days like these where I'm not happy with the number on the scale, I put on my sneakers, grab some headphones and go for a walk, listen to music and reflect, think, breathe. Let me be absolutely clear. I have never been on a super strict healthy diet in all the years (20+ so far) I've been on this journey. What I have done is try to make better food choices and reduce my intake of all food. As I've said before, I really don't like fruits or vegetables at all. Weight Watchers teaches you through their points system which items are better for you by calculating a points value for all food items. So my success has come from avoiding high point foods most of the time, portion control and exercise.

  I've always done some type of exercise even before I started on my journey. I guess I've always been an active person even when I was seriously overweight. At my highest weight, I went for walks outside while listening to music, bowled on a league and took country line dancing classes. I lived in an apartment for a few years which included a small gym and I would go there and try to use their equipment. I met a good friend that worked there in the evenings after returning from his duties at the Dover Air Force

Base. We are still friends today although he is hard to keep up with because he keeps moving to different states. I've always been intrigued by him. He was born in Chile, I met him in Delaware and visited him in California, Illinois and Washington. He lives in Texas now, but I haven't visited him there yet. Before I started my journey, I did some research, talked to people I worked with and tried a lot of different things. I've known people that have had their stomach stapled, lapband, bariatric and other surgeries to lose weight. I know one person that purposely gained weight in order to qualify for one of these surgeries. I know a couple people who have been successful after having one of these surgeries and one person who gained most or all of the weight back a few years after the surgery.

    I know a neighbor who was not fat that flew to Mexico to have some type of weight loss procedure and now is unbelievably thin. I say do whatever is going to work for you. I thought about all of these options before I started my journey, but I decided I wanted to do it through diet and exercise. I swear I have to do everything the hard way. I had reasons such as even at my highest weight I wasn't fat enough to

Keep It Off

qualify. I guess that was a blessing. It didn't make sense to me to gain more weight to qualify. Also, some of the restrictions after some of those procedures didn't sound good to me. Like no carbonated drinks afterwards?! Last time I checked, Diet Pepsi is carbonated. Or no sugar afterwards? Um ice cream, cookies, donuts, muffins, and all types of chocolate have sugar in them. Cake, cupcakes, candy bars, candy, etc!

Laugh! It's Medicine for the Soul
Humor and sarcasm are huge parts of my life. My family can make the most of any situation no matter how unpleasant or find something to laugh or be sarcastic about too. One of my favorite family stories came from preparing for my grandfather's funeral. We were all devastated when my grandfather died. He and my grandmother had been married over 50 years, lived in the same house my entire life and were the leaders of our family. Strong and true, always there for all of us.

So we were all at my grandparents house–me, my dad, my sister, my aunt, two uncles and my grandmother. My grandmother decided she wanted to bury my grandfather in pajamas and a robe. So my grandmother started bringing robes out of their bedroom into the living room where we were all sitting. The first one she brought out was a cream-colored long terry cloth robe. My uncle said no, I hate that one. The second one she brought out was a short burgundy silk robe with black trim. My dad said no, Hugh Heffner. My other uncle said: coming from a man wearing a Freddie Kruger sweater. We all looked over and yep, my dad was wearing a sweater that looked just like Freddie Kruger! The third one she brought out was a long green plaid and we all agreed that was the one. Then someone said, maybe my aunt, what about underwear? Someone said tighty whities. I said well he could go commando and my other uncle said what's commando and we all said none—no underwear at all. So during a sad time we all still found a way to be sarcastic and laugh.

> No great story starts with, "I was eating a salad."

Keep It Off

I also love to watch stand up comedians and comedy movies. My favorite back in the day was Eddie Murphy. These days it's Gabriel Iglesias (Fluffy) and Leanne Morgan for stand up. For movies, Jim Carrey and Melissa McCarthy are my favorites.

Do Not Shame Yourself in Any Way at Any Time
Shaming yourself is never the answer. As I fly home from a Tuesday through Thursday business trip to Chicago, I could focus on coulda, woulda, shoulda. I could focus on all the overeating I did. I could focus on all the exercise I didn't do. Instead I'm focusing on how much fun I had, how great it was to see and connect with people I only get to see a couple times a year if I'm lucky. I'm focussing on getting back on my program as soon as this plane lands. I will not overeat or make bad food choices for dinner tonight and will go to Zumba class. I did overeat on this trip. Tuesday night we went out to dinner for my 35th service anniversary and I did eat at one meal an arepa, empanada, flatbread, flank steak, potatoes, warm donuts with chocolate drizzle, chocolate cake and gelato. It was delicious!

Wednesday I did have breakfast at the Embassy Suites. I ate a one egg ham and cheese omelet, dry wheat toast, a few breakfast potatoes and a small double chocolate muffin. They got me a huge beautiful and delicious cake for my 35th service anniversary which I ate a huge piece of. I did eat two small pieces of thin pizza and a chocolate chip cookie for lunch. We did go out to dinner and I did eat what seemed like two full baskets of chips & salsa and one pork tamal. Today I tried to reel it in. I had the same breakfast as the day before minus the muffin and less breakfast potatoes, no lunch and grilled chicken and pita chips for dinner. I could beat myself up and go into a tailspin or whatever, but why? I thoroughly enjoyed the food and the activities.

I am accountable and acknowledge what I choose to do. Tomorrow is a new day. Let it go. Move on. Look forward. Start again. If you do have to look back, focus on any positive thing you can think of. I did meet my minimum step count each day. I did take the stairs instead of the elevator the whole time. I did drink water each day. I did try to track my food and drink intake. I did eat the thin pizza instead of the

Keep It Off

Chicago deep dish. I didn't get any Nerds candy even though it was right there in front of me the whole time.

On September 29, 2023 I made a conscious decision to lose and/or fail my 422nd consecutive daily step streak. I had 6,009 of my 12,650 daily step goal. It had been a long day. My son and I took the redeye to Philadelphia to surprise my dad for his 75th birthday. We went out to lunch at the Smyrna Diner in Delaware, hung out at my dad's, went to Costco to get a cake, went out to dinner to celebrate my dad's birthday, and hung out at my dad's some more. We made plans for a group of us to go to the Natural History Museum Smithsonian in Washington, D. C. the next day at 9:30 am. It was after 10 pm and I had been awake for over 34 hours. It would have taken me over 40 minutes to walk my remaining 6,641 steps so I decided it was okay to lose my step streak and go to bed instead. As much as my step streak meant to me as well as all of my goals, routines and consistency, I decided to let my step streak go for the rest of the weekend and just focus on enjoying and spending time with my family. And you know what, it was awesome.

If You Fail, Start Again

By the time I was on my flight back to Salt Lake City, my mind was already back in the right space. I restarted my daily step goal that day. I stayed within my Weight Watchers points that day. I went to Zumba that night. After overeating, barely exercising, and wondering how much weight I might have gained on that trip, I got right back into my routines and back on all my goals. I did not regret the decisions I made—right or wrong. I really wasn't disappointed that I gave up my step streak like I thought I would be. I enjoyed so much yummy food: chicken and dumplings, bread, steak, mashed potatoes, birthday cake, ice cream cake, chips and dip, buffalo chicken pizza, pepperoni pizza, and a hot fresh soft pretzel, but it was okay. Then I refocused. And I learned a new activity that I really enjoyed: corn hole. Maybe we could play it as a family when we got home?

I know so many people that say they want to lose weight and/or start an exercise routine. Sometimes they try and succeed for a while, but fall right back after a few months or weeks. I know and see so many people at Zumba and the gym that are there getting a workout, but for the most part do not look more fit or slimmer. They are putting in the effort or some effort. They have some intentions, but they are just not getting there.

If you take time off from exercise, when you get back to it, it's like starting over and it doesn't take much to feel that way. If I go on vacation for a week, when I return to my Zumba classes, I have to rebuild my endurance. I sweat more than usual and after a class or two I will feel sore. I have great endurance and don't feel sore if I'm consistent with my exercise. Recently I had to stop my Zumba classes for four weeks after having neck surgery. And trust me when I say I didn't want to because I love it and I knew what it would be like when I returned. I've been back at it for 4 weeks and I'm just about back to my usual self, but during many classes I've had to take breaks or I was sweating profusely. Many days many body parts were/are sore and my feet have been hurting bad most days.

> I left Zumba in the worst mood, said no one ever.

If you ever have to take a break from your regular exercise routine, you may go through this readjustment period. The same is true when you try a new type of exercise working muscles that you haven't worked before or in a new way. Maybe even muscles you didn't even know you had. An example that always surprises me because I exercise very regularly (walking 5 miles a day minimum, Zumba for an hour at least 4 days a week, hiking) is when I go to the office once a month and take the stairs to the third floor. I am seriously huffing and puffing by the time I get to the top?

If You Fail Again and Again, Figure Out What's Holding You Back

What is holding them back? What is holding you back? Do you not know how to get started? Do you not understand that it's a lifestyle change with a long term commitment? Is it something else? There are some sayings which seem cliche, but I find them to be true: You can do anything you put your mind to. I would say that what held me back was partially a lack of knowledge. I mean I'm not stupid. Eating ice cream and cookies or a massive quantity of anything is not good. And everyone knows the basic formula to lose weight: burn more calories than you take in. But what I didn't know and learned from Weight Watchers is based on my height, weight, gender and age, how many points, based on calories, saturated fat, sugar, and protein I should be taking in each day. How much food my body really needs. And that was just the tip of the iceberg for me. I learned about food, exercise, measurements, substitutions. I've read and learned so many things over the years and I continue to read, learn, grow, research, and try new things.

Some friends and family have shared their desire to lose weight and/or get fit and I listen and if asked, offer suggestions. I do wonder what is holding them back. What I have personally found is that I was eating too much of the wrong things and not moving my body enough. If you learn about food, make better food choices or at least less of the not so good food choices or both and find ways to get your body moving more you will be successful. Maybe the people I see or talk to are just not ready? I understand. I wasn't ready for a long time. Maybe they don't know how to start, where to start or what to start? I sincerely want to help everyone and anyone. How do I reach you? What can I do to help you?

Count Your Successes More Than Your Failures
Even after more than 20 years, I still have setbacks and disappointments. Somehow disappointments and successes motivate me, but in different ways. Success makes me want to keep going. Disappointments make me mad, sometimes pissed off and that just makes me work even harder. Right now I'm going through some things and I'm trying to figure it all out and reflect on my actions and make sure I'm being honest with myself. I'm in peri or full blown menopause. I take some supplements to help with the symptoms. A few pounds have crept up. I have been suffering with two pinched nerves in my neck causing pain in my left arm from my shoulder down to my hand. I've recently started two medications. One causes constipation and the other causes weight gain and increased appetite. Again, a few pounds have crept up. Did I mention I'm left handed? Recently I went on a business trip and

then a personal trip where I over ate and ate a lot of naughty food like cake.

But I came home and went right back to my eating and exercise plan. I went to Weight Watchers for my monthly weigh-in this past Saturday and had my worst weight in three years or more. Granted I'm still 13 pounds below my Weight Watchers goal of 125, but I'm 7 pounds higher than my all time personal goal of 105 and 100 pounds lost. And it was unexpected. Based on my home scale and what Weight Watchers scale usually reads, I expected to be at least a pound and a half less and in line with my last weigh-in but that was not the outcome. I have also been feeling very bloated and puffy in my stomach sporadically and not being regular if you get my point. I have also found myself overeating pita chips several times lately and kind of losing control.

No Excuses

But you know what? I've kind of adopted this motto of "No Excuses." I could blame it on menopause, the medication I'm taking, or say the Weight Watchers scale is not accurate, but "no excuses". Maybe some of these things are true and maybe they are not, but the bottom line is no excuses. I have to keep fighting for my goals. I could so easily accept all the excuses and just give in to it. Oh well, I have menopause so I'm going to gain weight. Oh well, the medication I'm taking causes weight gain and increased appetite so I'm going to gain weight. Oh well, the nerve pain in my arm hurts so bad, I have to stop exercising so I'm going to gain weight. Oh well. Nope! I have worked too long and hard to accept any of that! I am going to follow my eating and exercise plan that has made me successful up to now. I am going to stop overeating and getting out of control with pita chips. I am going to stop eating when I'm not hungry. I'm going to do a better job with portion control and staying within my Weight Watchers daily points. I am going to continue walking and doing Zumba when I'm in pain and it hurts. If the pain gets to be too much, I'll call the doctor again and see what they can do for me. I'm going to get my weight back to where I want it by next month and all months after! I didn't want to lose weight for just a little while. I wanted to lose it and keep it off forever.

Keep It Off

So I knew it was going to be a long term ongoing process. That I may take one step forward and two steps back many times and would have to find a way to be okay with that. I would have to be open to change (not my strong suite) and take many baby steps along the way. Just start! Just a baby step and another and then just keep going. I've made so many changes and tweaks over the years and I still have many to at least consider.

You have to be honest with yourself. Not hard on herself, just honest. You have to hold yourself accountable, but not too hard on yourself. Like me right now - I counted out one portion/serving of Stacy's pita chips, yes I did eat that serving and then go get the bag and get out of or lose control with eating them. Here's what accountability looks like to me: I acknowledged what I did and I logged in my Weight Watchers tracker a guess of how many points I think that was, I thought in my head that was not good and I also thought I'm going to try to do better tomorrow, and that's it! No dwelling on it, no thinking well I may as well go all out now, and definitely not beating myself up about it. How about another old cliche:

what's done is done. There is nothing I can do about it now unless I want a whole new issue to deal with. Be easy and kind to yourself.

Be Honest With Yourself: Reflect on What's Going On Inside of You

Reflection is a huge part of my journey. When I'm struggling, I spend a lot of time reflecting and analyzing the situation. I keep telling myself that my process has worked for over twenty years and it can continue to work. Maybe it just needs a tweak or some patience. Ha! Maybe I've gone slightly off course which has happened a few times and just need to reel myself back in. Or maybe current circumstances are contributing. I try to be honest with myself even if I don't like it.

Current circumstances: I have two pinched nerves in my neck causing severe pain in my left arm and shoulder. I may have to have surgery. I'm on a medication that has a huge list of possible side effects. A couple of them are increased appetite, weight gain and constipation. I've been overeating pita chips and on a few occasions gotten out of control with them.

Keep It Off

I've gained 5 pounds. I've lost my bathroom regularity. Is all or any of this related to the medication or am I just using that as an excuse or self fulfilling prophecy? I have also been feeling really bloated the last month or so. I have experienced this before and came up with a remedy and regimen that has worked for a couple years, but maybe not anymore? I am 55 now. Maybe it's menopause? Or maybe it's the ridiculous amount of Diet Pepsi I've been drinking? Maybe it finally caught up with me?

Is it my hormones, IBS, medication? Is my body going through some changes or adjustments? I don't really know exactly what is going on, but I've got my eyes wide open. I'm observing everything and ready to make some adjustments as needed. I do not want to put on any more weight! I'm not even hungry at meals or when I'm overeating! Is it stress? All I could say was I would stay the course. Take one day at a time. Work on each issue and try to make it better. Work on it until I fix it. I had stopped myself from overeating the pita chips, had counted out and eaten one portion and then went for the bag. I stopped myself and told myself no. That day, I was a success. I would see how tomorrow went and the next day, etc. I also didn't allow myself to have any snacks that day. I thought about it (the mind is strong), but told myself, 'I'm not even hungry so why eat a snack? Lunch is only two hours away.'

Keep It Off

Things that Inspire Me

I was looking through recipes, articles, and other things I had saved on my phone and came across an article from January 2023 called Weight Watchers Tips & Trips. I don't even remember saving the article, but it was refreshing and confirming to read an article written by someone else that has been on Weight Watchers as long as I have (20+ years). She writes about the same things I've been saying and writing about, as well as having long term success. Here are the tips and trips that were shared in the article:

- WW is a Lifestyle, not a Diet–it's the long game. Not a short term fix.
- Don't Deprive yourself–If you deprive yourself, you're not going to be able to sustain the lifestyle long term. Make sure you build in your favorite treats.
- Try not to eat after dinner / past 7pm–I personally do this to help with my IBS and because for weight loss you want to stop eating at least three hours before going to bed.

- Count everything you put in your mouth – eventually you will do this in your head, but when you are starting "on the program', you need to get a good sense of the points you are actually eating. You may not have to do this forever if you don't want to. After twenty years, I still manually track everything. I think it's key to my success.
- Take it one healthy choice at a time and repeat - just try to make your next choice a healthy one and then the next. This is a good long term strategy.
- If you fall off, get back on–Even if you're having a bad day, week, month or year and you overindulge and gain, just get back on track. If you mess up again, don't beat yourself up. Just keep getting back on track.
- Give yourself something to look forward to–tell yourself to wait until weigh-in day and then you can have whatever food or drink item you want if you still want it. Over time I've learned to reward myself with non-food items such as a new book or workout gear.

Keep It Off

- Exercise–Exercise makes you feel better and you'll gain muscle, which helps to burn fat and calories. Do what you can, even if it's walking around the block at first, and build up. But remember, it's only a small part of the equation. Please don't think because you work out you can eat a lot more. We often overestimate how much exercise we do or points we earn and underestimate how much we eat.
- The 80/20 Rule–when it comes to weight loss, food is the 80% and exercise is the 20%. I lost the first 40 of my 100 pounds doing hardly any exercise. I recently had neck surgery and could only walk for exercise. I only gained 3 pounds which is a miracle based on what I was eating.
- Don't be afraid to use all your points–On Weight Watchers, you get daily points and extra weekly points to use how and when you want. The points are there for you to use so go ahead and use them all! Daily and weekly points! You should still lose weight using all of your points if you're accurately counting everything you eat and drink.

- Only weigh yourself once a week– Weight fluctuates too much on a daily basis to get an accurate measure (due to water retention and other factors) if you weigh yourself more than once a week. If you gain, have a little cry (or a small pity party) then figure out why and get back to it! So you gained and it sucks, but it's a minor setback. Focus on how far you've come. Then get to work! Look at what you might have done to gain. Look at what you ate last week. Did you accurately count everything?
- Keep your eye on the prize–Losing weight is not sexy, it's not fun, nor is it easy, but it is damn well worth it. You know your weaknesses, so plan accordingly.
- If you're eating out, plan for it–If you're not familiar with the menu at the restaurant you're going to, you can access most menus online. So have a look, figure out the points, and plan what you will eat. You may want to save some points and indulge.
- Plan for potlucks too–If you're going to a potluck, always bring something you can eat as

well. Because I know myself, I do my best to avoid potlucks and buffets.
- Use seasonings–Everything bagel seasoning for example is 0 points and tastes great on so many things.
- Get yourself an air fryer–I don't have one and may need to take this advice!
- Cook normal food–But also make sure you keep healthy versions of your favorite food on hand so you're not tempted to indulge in high points food.

Diary of a Foodie

My mind is constantly running through random thoughts, observations, and reflections continually looking for self improvements or answers to my never-ending curiosity. Maybe your mind does the same thing or something similar? The following is a look into my mind and it may be a wild ride.

Saturday, September 10, 2023
Met a new goal today–365 consecutive days of walking at least 5 miles per day, 12,650 steps, burning 1600 calories, getting at least 60 minutes of exercise and at least 250 steps per hour twelve hours a day between 7 am to 7 pm. I want to keep going! How long can I go? It wasn't easy to get here for sure. On my way to Delaware at the beginning of June, I lost my FitBit in the airport and panicked. I had to backtrack and thankfully found it. I've had to get creative several times to keep the streak going. If you are with me at a restaurant and I'm a little longer in the bathroom than you think is normal or maybe you go to bed and still

hear me moving around hello! Goals! My previous record was 240 days.

I finally see myself thin. It took a really long time–several years–even though I've been the same size for at least 14 years. I realized before moving to Utah 16 years ago, the only real exercise I did was Curves for 30 minutes 3 days a week. Now I'm walking 5 miles per day, going to Zumba at least 4 days a week and hiking whenever I can fit it in and I love it!

It's 10:30 am. I got up, took my pills, did some chores and now I'm walking outside before it gets too hot and I'm thinking about what to eat. I'm not hungry at all but lunch is approaching. All I've had so far is a glass of water with ice and a piece of watermelon gum. Does that count? During the week (today is Saturday), I get up, have my breakfast with water at 6 am without thinking if I'm hungry or not. I take my lunch at 10:30 am because everyone is in a different time zone and schedule meetings around a normal lunch time but that's okay because by 10:30 I'm usually very hungry and maybe already had a snack. Then I have dinner between 5 - 6 pm before I go to my 7 pm Zumba and because I'm committed to not eating past 7 pm. At dinner I'm usually not hungry either but I eat anyway? Weekends are different but why and should they be? Maybe because I'm not working and don't get up at 5 am or earlier? Am I on to something here? Should I not eat until I feel hungry every day or should I get up and eat first on weekends like I do during the week? I've always heard breakfast is the most important meal of the day and you shouldn't skip meals. Is that true?

One of the things I love about the Zumba community is how the instructors and places volunteer their time and money when there is a person or family in need. Sometimes it's to raise money for a burial or an illness. They hold an event called a Zumbathon which is really like an extended Zumba class with multiple instructors and they ask for a minimum donation of $10.00. All proceeds go to the family in need. Zumbathons are even more fun than a regular Zumba class and for a good cause. Sometimes people donate items to raffle off or make food to sell. It's really amazing to see and participate in. And you wouldn't believe the crowd that comes out for it. Such a wonderful vibe!

Keep It Off

I also love when Erika Beltran (a Zumba Fitness Host, Zumba Instructor and Zumbawear Authorized Distributor in Utah) hosts an event called a Master Class where she brings in celebrities (such as Richi Angel, Mony Fuentes and Karina Rocha) local instructors and sells her Zumbawear. The events are so energized and fun!

Thanksgiving Day, 2023
Well here it is Thanksgiving Day and I have many things on my mind. Of course I'm thinking of all the many things I am thankful for and the list is very long. I'm thinking of friends, family, and acquaintances that are far away. I'm thinking of my friend Richard that's at the Macy's Thanksgiving Day parade in New York City fulfilling one of his bucket list items. I'm dreaming of one day marking that off my bucket list too. I'm thinking about how today represents a day of overeating and how to enjoy it but without a huge increase on the scale tomorrow. This basically applies to all holidays and celebrations. So first I make exercise a priority in my life and there is usually a morning Zumba class on holidays. I got up this

morning, had water, a chocolate protein shake, a fiber one brownie and went to Zumba. When I got home, I made chorizo with scrambled eggs and shredded cheese and half a skinny bagel with spray butter. I made sure to reach my daily step goal on my Fitbit. I got a little hungry in the early afternoon, so I had some pita chips. For Thanksgiving Dinner, I had one crescent roll, turkey breast, a little stuffing and mashed potatoes with gravy. It wasn't a lot but I was really full. I don't like pie so I had taken my favorite Crumbl chocolate cake cookie out of the freezer (they only offer this one twice a year) and planned to eat the whole thing as my dessert. Remember, I've been waiting for over 3 weeks to have a dessert since I was on the 21 day challenge, but I only ate half of the cookie. It was damn good, but I was too full to finish it and in the back of my mind I was thinking about how hard I worked on the 21 day challenge and how close I am to achieving my ultimate weight goal. I weighed

> Today I start my fast, everything I eat imma eat it fast as hell.

Keep It Off

105.8 this morning, So close! All in all, I don't think I did too bad today while still enjoying everything I ate. Let's see what the scale says tomorrow. I try to set myself up for success by watching what I eat before and after a holiday and making sure to go to Zumba before and after as well.

Friday, February 23, 2024
So, I had neck surgery a week ago. There are so many random thoughts going through my head that I want to capture here and I'm sure they will be all over the place, but there is an importance to all of them and a meaning from a support system, weight loss, fitness or general life perspective. Thursday night before my surgery, I was cleaning, organizing, shopping, making sure I got my daily steps in, and taking my last Zumba Class before going to the airport to pick up my best friend of over 40 years who offered to fly in and take care of me for the week following my surgery. I honestly had no idea what to truly expect. I'm terrible at being a patient or letting others take care of me and I knew there would be things I would not be able to do. And yes I did remind my friend of these things when

she offered to come. I love to be a hostess, make and buy things I know guests will like, cook, be a tour guide, etc. I knew this was going to be different from her usual visit, but I couldn't help being excited she was coming.

In case you ever have to prepare for a procedure using Hibiclens or other medical soap, it smells terrible, doesn't lather, is red and stains and I'm not sure why it is called soap. Special thank you to the lady that specifically told me not to get it on my face or private areas because it could burn. That was very important information that still makes me cringe when I think about it. We stayed up late talking, but had to get up early to be at the Surgery Center by 6 am. I had mixed feelings about the time, I mean good grief, I was hoping to sleep in at least a little bit and not get up even earlier than usual for work, but no. On the other hand, I was glad to get up, go and get it done and not have to starve all day or wait all day thinking and worrying about the surgery. After the surgery, my family and friend kept dozing off! They were exhausted! I should have been too! I never took a nap and stayed up all day until 10 pm that night and I couldn't stop talking! The surgery was 1 1/2 hours long, but must have been the best rest I had in 2 years dealing with the pain. They said I might have trouble swallowing for a few days after surgery, but it wasn't too bad.

I was overwhelmed by the number of family, friends, coworkers, and Zumba family that reached out to me to see how I was doing. I am truly blessed and appreciative. While my friend was here, it felt like I was on vacation with a much lighter itinerary. I did not take any of the prescription pain medicine they gave me. That doesn't mean I didn't have any pain. I have been taking muscle relaxers every night and Tylenol periodically. I've had a lot of discomfort in the bottom back of my neck and across my shoulders. Each day we went out for a little while to walk, but mostly binge watched shows based on books I've read, talked and ate. The most pain I had was at bedtime trying to get comfortable and first thing in the morning when I got up. I wasn't sure if I would be able to bathe myself or put my clothes on and I dreaded that. I don't like anyone to see me naked because I don't like how most of my body looks and the thought of how I wouldn't be able to do basic things! I was able to bathe and dress myself. My friend was here for a week and then flew home. Other than not going to Zumba on Saturday morning and needing help with the grocery shopping Sunday afternoon, the weekend was the same as usual.

But then Monday came and everything felt weird. Friday exactly one week after surgery, I started working back up to my hourly and daily step goals and I've been back on track since Sunday completely. While my friend was here, I didn't watch my diet very well and ate cookies, ice cream and other junk food although I haven't had much of an appetite lately so my portions were small. The day after she left, I started watching my diet closely again. One of my constant fears is gaining back the weight I've lost so if I gain 5 or more pounds I start to panic and buckle down. One of my concerns with having surgery was knowing that other than walking I would not be able to exercise for 4-6 weeks, which also brings back my fear of gaining weight. Also Zumba is my stress relief, therapy, getting out of the house, socialization, so how would I fill this gap?

Keep It Off

All of my regular routines were out the window. Did I mention that I am a creature of habit that enjoys routines and set schedules? Anyway, while my friend was here she kept me sane and occupied. She also helped me make sure I wasn't doing things I wasn't supposed to like bending and lifting. So although Monday came in feeling weird, I decided to embrace it and be positive. I decided to focus on the 3 R's (not reading, writing and arithmetic LOL) - relax, refresh and recover. Sunday night I made a list of things to do that I thought would last several days. Other than going to two stores, I had the list done by midday Monday.

So, now each day I try to add things to the list. Most days of the week I get up at 5 am or earlier, work 10 hours or so, breakfast at 6 am, lunch at 10:30 or 11 am, dinner between 5-6 pm, walk, read, write, Zumba, shower, in bed by 9 pm, asleep by 10 pm or so. So, Monday, I was up by 9 am, took a shower, went to Weight Watchers, had a fiber one bar in the car, stopped for gas and what I call a big soda and came home. I had a fried egg, skinny bagel and pita chips for lunch, and made some phone calls.

Throughout the day, I walked to get in my hourly and daily step goals. In between, I read and wrote. Booked a timeshare. Rescheduled some appointments. I had teriyaki chicken and rice for dinner. Watched a movie with my son. I was in bed by 10 pm. The whole week has been basically the same with a few minor variations. I've watched people at work be offered and take early retirement over the years. I've had the years of service required for a long time, but I'm not old enough yet. You have to be 55 and I'm not quite there yet, but I'm really close!

I've been praying for years that I can make it to at least 55 with Discover and continuing to do so. I've often wondered what in the world would I do with myself all day every day if I retired, but after being off work for the last two weeks now recovering from surgery, I think I could do it! I mean I've been taking it easy the last two weeks. I've only done light cooking, shopping and cleaning and for exercise, I've only been walking - no Zumba, hiking, gym, etc. and I've been able to find ways to fill my days with ease. I like to read a lot, but I don't normally watch TV shows. Only movies on weekends. The past two weeks I've watched a lot of shows and one movie based on books I've read: The Marsh King's Daughter, Will Trent, Fool Me Once, Home for Good and The Sandhamn Murders series.

One of my concerns with having surgery and only being able to walk for exercise and not take my 4-8 Zumba classes a week was gaining weight. I got down to my lowest weight ever right before surgery (104). It was exactly two weeks ago today that I had surgery and my weight has been fluctuating between 106-108. I'm okay with that. Two weeks from today, I will go to my post surgery follow-up where I hope to hear that I'm healing well and can return to my regular physical activity. I just need to hold my weight steady for two more weeks. I think I can do that. I am still having nerve pain in my left arm which is what the surgery in my neck was supposed to fix.

I talked to the nurse practitioner the other day and she said it could take a long time for the nerves to fully heal (up to 2 years) and the nerves were stretched along with the muscles during the surgery so everything is irritated right now. They put two spacers in and I'm supposedly half an inch taller! I'm a short girl so I'll take any half inch I can get! Anyway, I already feel like I have more energy than ever and I'm optimistic that the pain will go away and I'll be back out there killing it again soon!

Another concern I have post surgery is my hair. The last time I had surgery was about four years ago on my thumb. Several weeks after surgery, my hair started falling out when I washed it in the shower and when I brushed it. My hair got very thin for the first time in my life. I have always had thick, fluffy, unruly hair. I talked to my hair dude about it and he recommended a dietary supplement (Biotin which is good for nails, skin and hair) which I started taking immediately and still take every single day. I also ordered and used Ovation Cell Therapy hair and scalp treatment, shampoo and conditioner. Eventually my hair got thick again and has remained thick, but here I am two weeks post neck surgery and I'm wondering if it will happen again. I'm trying not to worry about it. Like in the past, I was able to resolve it. Only time will tell.

I've found myself backsliding on some of my goals from the 21 day challenge back at the end of

Keep It Off

October, primarily significantly reducing soda intake and stopping overeating pita chips. I did really well with these two goals as well as three others after the challenge for a couple months and then slowly but surely I started drinking more soda and overeating pita chips again.

    Right before my surgery two weeks ago, I was at my lowest weight ever, I haven't had much of an appetite (maybe because of the medication?) so I've skipped dinner occasionally when I was really busy, not really hungry and didn't have time to eat until about 9 pm which is too late for me. I try not to eat past 7 pm for weight loss and other reasons. So, my question after saying all of that is does it really matter that I am backsliding on these two things? In addition, I have also started eating candy again - Nerds and smarties. I had given up candy except a little around the holidays, but now here I am eating candy by the bag or box again at a time when I can't even do any exercise except walking to even attempt to burn it off! What am I doing and why am I doing it?! I'm not craving it! I'm not even hungry! I'm also drinking a lot less water. I need to reel myself back in. I think this speaks to how difficult it is to be on maintenance after weight loss and how easy it is to backslide on things. The key is to recognize there is an issue/backslide and reel it back in before you allow it to get too far. Maybe there are things I will always struggle with or at least more difficult to maintain or make the change stick. It would be so easy just to give in, but I've worked too hard to allow it.

My Heroes

Samantha Madsen

I think I've mentioned Samantha Madsen (Sam) who was an instructor at a gym I went to until it closed. She was previously a professional bodybuilder, has a Master's Degree in Exercise Physiology, Bachelor's in Exercise & Sports Science & Nutrition, owns Luxe Body Worx, I could go on and on about all of her amazing accomplishments as well as she's just an incredible person. Anyway, I joined her mailing list a few months ago after seeing her and buying some of her soaps and other products. She recently shared an article that resonated with me titled - Maintaining Bodyweight - My 7 Tips I Live By. Now I bet Sam hasn't ever been overweight, but her 7 tips are the same or similar to the tips I used to lose weight and use today to maintain my weight loss. When I read her article, I thought YES YES YES!!! And now let me share her full article here:

Hello beautiful!

I wanted to share with you what I have been doing for decades to maintain my body weight. This isn't about weight loss per se, but more about maintaining the weight you're at or, once you've arrived, the weight you might be working toward. Maintaining weight can be easy but like everything worthwhile in life, it comes with effort, habits, and discipline.

1. Drink plenty of water. This is my number one. Why? It truly takes at least 100 ounces of water intake a day to maintain optimal hydration. And if you're exercising or moving a lot, you need more. Most people walk around somewhat dehydrated. Dehydration negatively affects every system in the human biome. The nerve pathway that tells the brain you're hungry is the same nerve pathway that tells the brain you're thirsty. Sometimes, when you think you might want a snack, what you really need is a big drink of water. The only way to know how much water you're taking in is to measure it. Fill a 20 ounce bottle of water and ensure you empty it five times a day. Too simple.

Keep It Off

2. Weigh. Yes, you must get on a scale. A scale tells you where you're at and direction you're going, up or down. If you added a couple of pounds, you are informed and can make small changes to correct it. This is how you keep from gaining weight year after year. Weigh at the same time (or close to it) as you did the last time. In other words, don't weigh one day in the morning, and the next time at 2 in the afternoon. Weigh time should be relatively consistent. Personally, I weigh every morning. At minimum, once a week. There are some days when I don't want to get on the scale because maybe I ate a salty meal or I might have eaten badly. But what has avoidance ever done for anyone? Suck it up buttercup and hop on the scale. Not weighing is a demonstration in denial and avoidance. One day doesn't define you.

3. Eat until you're full (not stuffed). As soon as you feel full, stop eating. Full is not stuffed. Full is just comfortable. If needed, you could go for a walk afterward. You don't feel like sleeping or lounging. This requires discipline and practice. But, I promise, it does get easier. Fill your plate or bowl with what you might eat and most of the time, that's all you need.

Once you've mastered eating till full, and you overeat, you'll rarely do it again because of the discomfort. It's so empowering having this mastery over food.

4. Reduce sugar intake. Clearly eating sweets, pastries, and sweet dairy products makes maintaining weight very challenging. While steering clear of this type of food is beneficial, this isn't really what I'm talking about. Sugar lurks everywhere. Browse your pantry and look at the labels on salad dressings, spaghetti sauces, yogurt, condiments, seasoning sauces, fruit juices and the like. You'll be surprised where and how you are consuming sugar. Reduce sugar intake where you can, like buying low sugar or sugar free yogurt, making your own salad dressings, eliminating fruit drinks or fruit juices (better off eating the fruit), and comparing sauce labels to purchase the lowest sugar options (if it's one you must have). Regarding sweets, pastries, and sweet dairy products, eat minimally and only on occasion. Regular consumption is guaranteed weight gain.

5. Eat greens. Eat a big bowl of greens every day and top it with chopped vegetables of every variety. You can also drink your greens but not out of a bottle (too much added sugar). Make your own green drink at home using a high powered blender. I made a video sharing the ingredients and how I make this. I drink it four times per week. Eating greens not only makes you feel better and provides disease fighting foods, it also promotes good weight. If you're filling up on greens and vegetables, you're less likely to eat junk. On the days I drink my green drink, most of the time I'm still eating a bowl of greens.

6. Consistent exercise. Our bodies were meant to move. Not sit. Seven to nine hours is already spent in slumber. It doesn't matter what type of movement or exercise you do. Walking, cycling, lifting weights, jogging, dancing, group fitness classes, whatever. Just do something at least six days a week. Exercise burns calories, builds muscle, and improves balance. It makes you feel better. The American College of Sports Medicine (ACSM) recommends moderate-intensity exercise 30 min 5 days a week and vigorous-intensity exercise 20 minutes 3 days a week, or a combination. Research over the last decade has shown that the lack of exercise is as unhealthy as smoking cigarettes. Yes! Let that sink in.

7. Don't eat three hours before bed. We sleep better when our stomachs are not full or having to digest food while we sleep. After dinner, don't snack. It's more of a habit than being hungry. If you get a hankering for something, sip on low sugar hot chocolate or a flavored tea (don't add milk or cream). Consuming a small mint or chewing gum can help reduce cravings. If you must snack, choose a low calorie food like a small apple, a few celery or carrot sticks, a small bag of Skinny Pop popcorn, a boiled egg, or 1 to 2 TBSPs blanched nuts (any variety just not the salted or flavored kind). Not eating after dinner takes a bit of discipline and practice. However, this one thing can show dramatic results.

Consistency creates habits. Good habits feed success. These are my habits I've been doing for decades. Sure, do I eat a bowl of ice cream on occasion or a fat laden meal? Of course I do. I just don't do it all the time. Weighing every day lets me know where I'm at so that I can make the necessary adjustments before the situation becomes more challenging than I want it to be.

Keep It Off

I hope you've found this useful and helpful. Would love to know your own good habits and what you do that's helped you stay healthy.

Stay grounded in the things that matter, find ways to serve others, and share kindness wherever you are. Continue to rise, reach, and become.

Forever Your Champion, Samantha

Rachel Hollis

I love Rachel Hollis. She is open, direct and transparent. I relate to her and feel like I'm like her in so many ways. I listen to her podcasts on so many different topics. I flew back to Delaware to be with my friend for her kidney surgery and while I was there I started and finished Rachel Hollis's book Didn't See That Coming. It was amazing. I love her style of writing and how she just puts it out there! Anyway, while I was there with my friend and she was dealing with her surgery and her other illnesses, I was thinking here I am writing a book, how I wish I could help her, my mom, and other friends/family with their weight and fitness.

If I could just be relatable with my material like Rachel Hollis! When I read one of her books, I get sucked in and I don't want to stop. How can I make my book be like that and especially for my loved ones? I'm now reading her latest book and I've loved it since the first word - What if YOU Are the Answer? I also saved some more of her podcasts to listen to. Please join me and get on the Rachel Hollis band wagon! Maybe I should join her fan club? Wonder if she has one? I would love to talk to her just one time and go to one of her events. In all of her books she talks about going to therapy and how valuable it has been to her. I have finally decided to try it in 2025. I have some healing I need to do and some things I need to clear out. I went to my first session this week and I will say it was very painful during the session and the day after, but since I feel so good!

I saw this Meme/Quote on Facebook: Helping one person might not change the world, but it might change the world for one person. When I started out writing this book, my goal was if I could help at least one person get on their journey to lose weight and/or be physically active, I would be a success, but if I can't

Keep It Off

reach those closest to me, how will I be able to reach other people I don't even know? How do I reach you? That's my purpose in writing this book, and I can honestly say that Rachel Hollis was a big inspiration for me.

Case Studies

As I was writing this book, I thought a lot about all the weight loss strategies and fitness activities I tried for years before I settled into what worked best for me - Weight Watchers, Zumba, hiking. That is all shared in the preceding chapters. Then I was thinking about you, the readers, and what if my strategies or activities sounded good, but didn't really suit you? Or you were thinking, 'I wish she talked about other options for weight loss and fitness'? So, I phoned four amazing friends who have traveled a different path with similar results and asked them if they would let me interview them about their journeys. This chapter is the result. In it you'll read about two very different weight loss and two very different fitness journeys. I hope that their incredible tips and experiences may be helpful to you.

Weight Loss Journey #1–Wade Baldwin
Hi, my name is Wade Baldwin. I was born and raised in Utah. I met Kristie while working at Discover

Keep It Off

Financial Services about 24 years ago and we have been friends ever since.

For many years, I tried different diets to lose weight such as Atkins (low carb), counting calories, Keto, etc. but wasn't able to keep the weight off. Family events, holidays and vacations were very difficult for me. My mom was an amazing cook. During these times, it was very difficult to be good with my food intake. When I got to my heaviest, I was 350 pounds (although I am 6' 3" tall). I was working and going to school and not exercising at all. If I did try to workout, I would be in a lot of pain due to continuous neck and back injuries and worried I would injure myself. I was thrilled to go to Leatherby's (an ice cream place) that had a Mexican Restaurant inside as it's my favorite food. I had no portion control at all. I was embarrassed getting on my friend's ATV or having to buy 2 seats on an airplane. I was literally rolling out of bed, disgusted with myself, couldn't keep up with my small son and had another one on the way. I was basically a food addict and my 'you're full switch' was broken. I knew I had to do something. I said this is it and I was desperate to do something.

I heard about bariatric surgery at work, but at the time didn't think or consider going that route to shed the weight. I ended up deciding to pursue gastric bypass surgery. You have to go to an introductory class, talk to someone about all the things you have tried for at least six months prior and meet a specific BMI. You have to go into it thinking it's a life cycle change or you will not be successful so that's what I did. After the surgery, your stomach is so small. You can only eat very small quantities while slowly reintroducing foods back into your daily diet. My 'you're full switch' started working again and most of the time I did not feel hungry due to the reduced size of my stomach, but I still had cravings. Also after the surgery, you have to eat kind of like a Keto diet which was not too hard for me as I was very familiar with Atkins. With gastric bypass, you need to avoid sugar. You will learn about dumping syndrome (food or sugar moves too quickly) and if you eat something high in sugar such as ice cream, you will get the sweats and shakes and begin to feel very weak.

With gastric bypass, I lost up to 165 pounds. Reaching your target weight is not the end! You still

Keep It Off

have to work to maintain. I weigh myself once a week and generally stay between 195-200 pounds. If I start to see myself going above 200 pounds ('the line' for me is 210), I buckle down, bring back the consistency to get back to my box of what I can/can't do and what is acceptable. Everybody has to decide what their 'line' is. .

    The hardest part of my journey was asking for and seeking help. Some people find value in the support groups, but that really isn't/wasn't my thing. The easiest part for me was giving up desserts. I enjoy them, but can forgo them. Being consistent, accountable and tracking my intake has helped me keep the weight off. My health has improved, I'm more in tune with my body, I can be more active, I know my limits, I'm better able to handle my chronic back issues and support my family. I never want to go back to where I was! I'm mostly happy with how I look now. I mean the extra skin doesn't go away of course.

Tips/Thoughts/Quotes/Suggestions:
- Find your way and forgive yourself!

- Don't be self punishing. Just regroup and move forward.
- It's not a diet, it's a mindset/lifestyle change.
- You can't do it for others. You have to do it for yourself. This is the same with any addiction. I did it for myself when I quit drinking and when I had weight loss surgery.

These days, I enjoy spending time with my wife and three sons. We love to travel within Utah and all over camping, hiking, scuba diving and other outdoor activities. Thanks to the surgery I decided to get, I now feel lighter, healthier and more confident.

Weight Loss Journey #2– Diana Munoz Coronado
Hi, my name is Diana Munoz Coronado. I was born and raised in Ecuador. I studied Social Work at Brigham Young University - Idaho. I am a Family Consultant at Catholic Community Services of Utah. I became a social worker because I love and deeply care about all people. I want to be an example for my family and others. I met Kristie about four years ago while I was teaching Zumba classes at The Nutrition in

Keep It Off

Kearns Utah. I am married and have three young sons and two dogs.

All of my pregnancies were high risk. With my first son, I gained 50 pounds, but was able to lose it. With my second son, I gained 25 pounds, but wasn't able to lose it. With my third son, I gained 60 pounds and during the pregnancy I had to take steroids. I tried everything - mediterranean diet, Herbalife, intermittent fasting to name a few. I would lose 15 pounds, but would then get stuck. I got depressed and was facing being a diabetic. I also didn't like what I saw in the mirror. I knew I had to do something. I went to a nutritionist and started a very strict diet. For 3 months I could only eat vegetable soup and I was going to Zumba every day. I lost 50 pounds! The nutritionist taught me how to eat–protein first, then vegetables, carbs last and drink a lot of water. It was really hard, but I am so proud of myself. I've lost 85 pounds! After losing 85 pounds, I went back to the doctor, did all the tests and everything came back perfect!

My husband has always been my biggest supporter! He has always told me and made me feel beautiful no matter my size. My mom has supported me throughout as well even when she was trying to feed me! My husband supported me during my strict diet and when I decided to get my tummy tuck and boobs adjusted (not enlarged). After losing 85 pounds, everything was saggy. I did a lot of research in advance and went to different places with the best doctors to use a machine to tighten my skin, get my tummy tucked and my boobs adjusted. The tummy tuck was not painful, but the boobs were very painful!

I'm still the same person I always was, but I have more self esteem and energy now and I love how I look. I would still like to lose another 20 pounds, but I'm really just trying to maintain what I lost. I try to be good as much as I can and follow what the nutritionist taught me–make good choices, make sure what you're eating is worth it. I have mostly cut sugar from my regular daily diet. The only sugar I have on a regular basis is in my daily coffee. I'm so happy to be able to buy clothes that I love now instead of having to buy what I could find that would fit!

Exercise has been a huge part of my success and also comes easy to me because I love it so much! I run and continue to increase the number of miles I am able to run. I teach and attend Zumba classes regularly.

Tips/Thoughts/Quotes/Suggestions:
- Believe in yourself! Don't give up! You can do it! Keep trying!
- It's not a diet, it's a lifestyle!
- Use a small plate! Cut a small piece and you will probably be satisfied.
- Allow yourself a cheat day.
- If there are things you can do for yourself that will make you feel more confident and better about yourself, you should do it!

These days, I enjoy spending time with my husband and three sons and teaching Zumba classes.

Fitness Journey #1 – Samantha Madsen
Hi, my name is Samantha Madsen. I was born and raised in Utah. I'm currently the owner of Luxe Body Worx and a Fitness Instructor at Vasa – a chain of gyms in the Western US.

I have been very active my entire life. Our family trips and vacations always included outdoor activities. I have always been very athletic, muscular and strong. In Elementary School, I participated in running events. In Junior High School, I participated in gymnastics and track. In High School, I did gymnastics, track and swimming, and started long distance running my sophomore year.

I was working at Salt Lake International Airport and happened to be in a dress. I saw a poster of bodybuilders and at the same time someone saw me and said with calves like that you should be a bodybuilder! The poster and the comment set me on a new path! I started school on the Business track but didn't finish it because I soon realized it was not for me. I went back to school and now hold a Bachelor's Degree in Exercise & Sports Science, a Master's Degree in Exercise Physiology with Minors in Nutrition and Chemistry. I started lifting weights and joined the YMCA. I started working with a coach in 1982, Dennis Madsen, who later became my husband. I was in my first bodybuilding competition in 1983 and took 3rd place. I competed in one Powerlifting competition where I had the 7th best bench in the country and won the state title! The following year I won the bodybuilding competition. I was the only person in Utah (male or female) to win the State Championship in both powerlifting and bodybuilding. To achieve this, I had to learn how to diet and how to eat. I had to adopt a very serious, healthy and disciplined diet. I ate smart, high calorie, never lost my menstrual cycle and got my BFP (body fat percentage) to 4%!

People say they do not have time, but you can find time for all the things you are committed to achieving. I had to create a spreadsheet to help me as I was going to school, working, working out and competing at the same time.

I have always been self-driven and motivated. My Why: The possibility of developing an illness or disease continually motivates me to eat better. I often read medical journals. Eating healthy makes me feel better, keeps my sugar and cholesterol where it should be and more available to help others. I eat pizza and ice cream from time to time, but not every day. (All things in moderation. Don't deprive yourself! Don't stuff yourself!) I stay away from sodas as carbonation causes so many issues. I stay away from potato chips. I keep trigger foods out of the house. Chocolate chip cookies are my weakness (I can't believe she has the same exact weakness that I have!) and if they are in the house I will eat them. It's hard, but I strive to be consistent with clean and healthy eating.

Tips/Thoughts/Quotes/Suggestions:
- Nothing tastes as good as fitness feels!
- A sedentary lifestyle is as bad as smoking cigarettes!
- It doesn't matter where you are. Everyone starts somewhere so just do something. 1 small change at a time.
- You have to make a realistic commitment to start. Make it yours and own it!
- A lot of people need a buddy or an external motivation.
- Find and do an exercise that you love.
- Being healthy and losing weight isn't easy. Set yourself up for success mindfully and on purpose!

Keep It Off

- Use the scale at least once a week.
- Books: Joel Fuhrman–Eat to Live and David Kessler–The End of Overeating.

These days, I teach classes, still lift 6 days a week because I love it, bike, hike and ski staying active and healthy.

Fitness Journey #2 – Cirilo Albino DeJesus
Hi, my name is Cirilo Albino DeJesus. I was born and raised in Mexico City. I do all different types of construction for homes and businesses. I met Kristie at Jordan Valley Athletic Club about 10 years ago at fitness classes we both attended. Unfortunately, Jordan Valley Athletic Club closed about 5 years ago.

When I was about 30 (15 years ago) I recognized that I had a problem with alcohol drinking way too much and decided it was time to stop. After I quit drinking I was bored and didn't have anything in common with my friends/drinking buddies anymore. My dad always told me you should keep your mind and body busy so I decided to join the gym.

When I first started going to the gym, I felt lost because I didn't know what to do for my workouts. I was shy to go to the classes offered and thought they were just for women because that's who I saw in the classes. I decided to start going to the classes anyway, tried them and loved them and had some incredible instructors that taught me so much–boot camp, total body conditioning (TBC), spinning, Zumba, power flex, high intensity interval training (HIIT), and tabata. The instructors motivated and pushed me and I pushed myself. I found that exercising in group classes is motivating and makes me push myself as well. I also enjoy the connections you make at the gym with people that have the same or similar fitness goals. It's a true blessing to have incredible instructors, but it also makes it difficult when you experience less incredible instructors. As with many things in life, take the good things you learn and carry them with you. Keep your motivation and don't allow a less than good instructor or experience hinder you from keeping to your journey and working towards your goals.

Keep It Off

Exercise is the best thing you can do for your body. There are so many benefits to working out such as:
- It's the best therapy.
- Helps remove stress.
- Gives you more energy.
- Gives maintenance to your muscles.
- Working out makes you feel good. If you are sad, mad, happy, lost your job, lost your partner, GO TO THE GYM!
- Makes you focus on maintaining a good weight.
- Helps you live longer
- Helps you avoid medical conditions such as diabetes, high blood pressure, heart disease, cholesterol to name a few.

I'm not yet satisfied with how I look and I think I can do better! When I'm at the gym, I enjoy sharing my experience and knowledge with others about preparing for workouts and recovering from workouts with supplements and protein shakes and how to do the workouts correctly without injuring yourself.

Tips/Thoughts/Quotes/Suggestions:
- I don't lift weights, weights lift me!
- Love yourself! If you do, you will want to take care of your body.

These days, I attend Studio Red classes, do my own weight lifting and fitness routines and boxing at Vasa (a chain of gyms in the Western US) as many times a week as I can based on my work schedule. As soon as I walked into the West Valley Centennial Vasa, I knew I belonged there and thought, this is my place and my people! Sometimes I have to work far from home or long hours and I have to miss going to the gym. My job is also very physical which helps me maintain daily body activity each day. I like to bike, hike, travel and go on spontaneous adventures staying active as much as possible. I also enjoy relaxing and recovering when I'm not working or working out.

Keep Going, Keep Coming Back

Some days I still feel like I'm just figuring this out.

Yes, I've lost 100 pounds.

Yes, I've kept it off.

Yes, I've done the work.

But that doesn't mean I don't still have to fight for it every single day especially when I'm staring down a chocolate chip cookie.

Because let's be honest: this whole thing? It's not a before-and-after story. It's a before, a during, a setback, a comeback, a re-do, a "who cares let's eat pizza," a "get it together, girl," and a *start again on Monday* story.

And then do it again.

The truth is, weight maintenance is not the destination. It's the vehicle that lets you show up in your life the way you want to. That lets you feel strong and free and present. That lets you go for a hike without stripping off all your clothes halfway up a mountain. That lets you play corn hole and eat mashed potatoes and still love yourself the next morning.

Because you know what? That is success.

It's not a perfect body. It's not a magic number. It's not six days of Zumba in a row or going thirty days without Diet Pepsi (though if you ever see me do that, please check for a pulse).

It's deciding you're worth the effort—again and again. Even when the scale won't budge. Even when your stretchy pants feel tight. Even when someone brings donuts to work and your brain short-circuits.

It's learning that consistency doesn't mean perfection. It means you come back. Every time.

I've learned that setbacks don't mean failure. They mean you're human. And being human is not the problem—it's the whole point.

This book is not a blueprint. It's not a 30-day plan. It's not "the secret."

It's just the truth about what worked for me. What I figured out over time. What I'm still figuring out. What I messed up, what I learned, and what I laughed through.

Keep It Off

My hope is that somewhere in here, something made you feel less alone. Like maybe you don't have to do it perfectly. Like maybe you can start over without starting from scratch. Like maybe you can stop trying to earn your worth and just take care of the body and life you already have.

And if you got anything out of this, I hope it's this:

You can do hard things. You are not behind. You don't need to hate yourself to change yourself. And the most important weight to lose? Is the guilt and shame you've been carrying.

This isn't the end. It's just the start, the beginning... keep going.

Keep showing up. Keep saying no to the Oreos. Keep being a badass in your own life and mind.

And if you ever feel like quitting?

Come back.

You already know the way.

About the Author

Kristie Williams is mother to Sean Williams, long-time member of Weight Watchers, long-time employee of Discover Financial Services and lover of Zumba. She lives in Salt Lake City, Utah. In her free time, she loves to read, hike, travel, eat and talk.

The before picture you see below shows Kristie at the very beginning of her journey at 205 pounds, holding the son who inspired her to change.

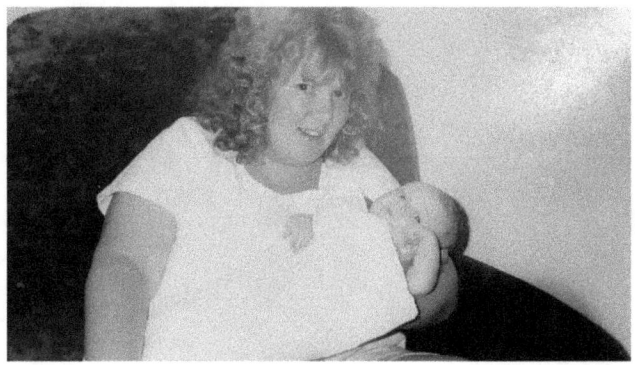

The recent photo below shows her on a Mother's Day hike with her son–with 14 years of healthy weight and

Keep It Off

fitness and counting! From day one with her son to today, Kristie turned her 'why' into a healthier, stronger life. Her hope is that she can help you do the same.

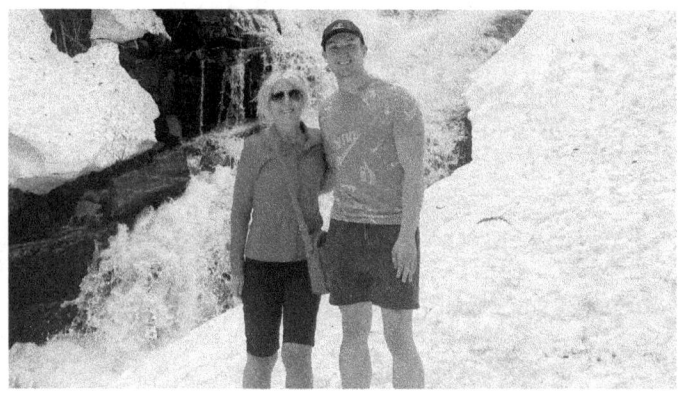

Suggested Books & Businesses

Books by Author Rachel Hollis
Girl, Wash Your Face
Girl, Stop Apologizing
Didn't See That Coming
What if YOU Are the Answer

Businesses
1. Luxe Body Worx https://luxebodyworx.com
2. Ole Nutrition 3360 S 5600 W, West Valley City, UT 84120
3. The Nutrition in Kearns 4081 W 5415 S, Kearns, UT 84118
4. ZW Zumba Wear Authorized Distributor in Utah Erika Beltran

www.ingramcontent.com/pod-product-compliance
Lightning Source LLC
Chambersburg PA
CBHW051532020426
42333CB00016B/1885